Strong Women, Strong Backs

MIRIAM E. NELSON, PH.D.

Friedman School of Nutrition Science
and Policy, Tufts University

with

LAWRENCE LINDNER, M.A.

◈

A PERIGEE BOOK

Strong Women, Strong Backs

EVERYTHING YOU NEED
TO KNOW TO PREVENT,
TREAT, AND BEAT
BACK PAIN

A PERIGEE BOOK
Published by the Penguin Group
Penguin Group (USA) Inc.
375 Hudson Street, New York, New York 10014, USA
Penguin Group (Canada), 90 Eglinton Avenue East, Suite 700, Toronto, Ontario M4P 2Y3, Canada
(a division of Pearson Penguin Canada Inc.) • Penguin Books Ltd., 80 Strand, London WC2R 0RL,
England • Penguin Group Ireland, 25 St. Stephen's Green, Dublin 2, Ireland (a division of Penguin
Books Ltd.) • Penguin Group (Australia), 250 Camberwell Road, Camberwell, Victoria 3124, Australia
(a division of Pearson Australia Group Pty. Ltd.) • Penguin Books India Pvt. Ltd., 11 Community Centre,
Panchsheel Park, New Delhi–110 017, India • Penguin Group (NZ), 67 Apollo Drive, Rosedale,
North Shore 0745, Auckland, New Zealand (a division of Pearson New Zealand Ltd.) • Penguin Books
(South Africa) (Pty.) Ltd., 24 Sturdee Avenue, Rosebank, Johannesburg 2196, South Africa

Penguin Books Ltd., Registered Offices: 80 Strand, London WC2R 0RL, England

While the authors have made every effort to provide accurate telephone numbers and Internet addresses at
the time of publication, neither the publisher nor the author assumes any responsibility for errors, or for
changes that occur after publication. Further, the publisher does not have any control over and does not
assume any responsibility for author or third-party websites or their content.

PRINTING HISTORY
G. P. Putnam's Sons hardcover edition / September 2006
Perigee trade paperback edition / September 2007

Perigee trade paperback ISBN: 978-0-399-53360-0

The Library of Congress has cataloged the G. P. Putnam's Sons hardcover edition as follows:

Nelson, Miriam E.
Strong women, strong backs : everything you need to know to prevent, treat, and beat back pain /
Miriam E. Nelson with Lawrence Lindner.
p.   cm.
Includes index.
ISBN 0-399-15375-6
1. Backache—Treatment.   2. Women—Health and hygiene.   3. Women—Diseases.   I. Lindner,
Lawrence.   II. Title.
RD768.N45   2006   2006043221
617.5'64—dc22

PRINTED IN THE UNITED STATES OF AMERICA

10   9   8   7   6   5   4   3   2   1

PUBLISHER'S NOTE: Neither the publisher nor the authors are engaged in rendering professional advice or services to the individual reader. The ideas, procedures, and suggestions contained in this book are
not intended as a substitute for consulting with your physician. All matters regarding your health require
medical supervision. Neither the authors nor the publisher shall be liable or responsible for any loss or
damage allegedly arising from any information or suggestion in this book.

Penguin Group (USA) Inc. is not associated with the StrongWomen™ Program.

For Mason

An Important Caution

◈

The advice given in *Strong Women, Strong Backs* is based on extensive scientific research. This book contains instructions and safety precautions. It is essential that you read them carefully. Some exercises are inappropriate for individuals with poor back health, back pain, or other medical conditions.

This book is not intended to replace the services of a health care provider who knows you personally. An essential element of taking responsibility for your health is having regular checkups and working in partnership with medical professionals.

If you are under treatment for back problems or any other medical condition—or if you suspect you might need such care—you must discuss this program with your doctor before you begin.

Contents

◈

Preface: Another Good Reason to Exercise

───────◆───────

In the twenty-plus years that I and other exercise physiologists have been studying the effects of strength training, aerobics, and other types of physical activity, more and more has come to light about just how beneficial movement is. You don't need to be a researcher to be aware of all the well-established proof that exercise offers the body myriad bonuses. As so many reports in newspapers and magazines and on television now frequently and consistently make clear, exercise improves strength; protects the heart, lungs, and the rest of the cardiovascular system; helps ward off osteoporosis; decreases the risk for diabetes; is a pillar of any weight-control effort; literally lifts depression; decreases the pain of arthritis; may play a role in staving off Alzheimer's disease and other types of dementia; and pushes back the creeping frailty associated with aging.

But ironically, one important benefit of physical activity is often not highlighted in the press. Exercise protects the back—the source of pain for so many people at so many different points in their lives. There is hardly a woman alive, in fact, who at some point has not "thrown out" her back one way or another, had to sleep on the floor, *couldn't* sleep, couldn't reach, couldn't go to work or attend to other obligations because the pain in her back wouldn't let her. Yet the research is solid and strong: regular exercise decreases back pain and even keeps it from coming on, or at least keeps it from getting as bad as it can. I have seen this over and over again—from women who have participated in the many exercise studies we have conducted at Tufts University as well as from women all over the world who have participated in community exercise programs.

In addition to my professional perspective, I am personally aware of exercise's positive effect on the back, since, as this book will detail, I had chronic back problems for many years and also know just how relieving to the spine the right kinds of physical activity can be. Now I want to bring the proof to you.

With the right exercises *and* the right attention given to other aspects of lifestyle—sleep patterns, the ergonomics of your work space and your home, how you handle stress—there is much you can do to ameliorate back pain and even keep it from recurring. That is, pain in your spine is not a given. You are not stuck with it. By making changes in how you live, you can truly keep your back from getting in the way of living your life to the fullest.

PART 1

◆

New Ways to Understand Back Pain

◆

CHAPTER 1

You Are Not Alone: Most People Experience Back Pain

When I was in the sixth grade, my friend Barbie (yes, that was her real name) challenged me to a gymnastics contest. It was recess, with no teachers around, and the test we devised was to see how high we could dive-roll over boxes that we placed on a mat—sort of like starting a somersault while jumping into the air and then rolling over the boxes as we stacked them higher and higher.

Each time we completed a dive we added more boxes, and even though in my memory they stacked up really high, they couldn't have stood much over a foot or two. Still, after numerous dives, my arms started to tire, until I reached the point that they couldn't support me through a dive and I landed flat on my head.

I felt myself crumple—and my back felt strange enough that I knew not to move. My friend went to get a teacher, who thought I simply had the wind knocked out of me and just told me to take some deep breaths. But my back still didn't feel right.

The school called an ambulance, and the X-rays at the hospital showed that I had crushed three of my vertebrae—bones that support the back. It was right in the middle of my spine, the thoracic region.

I had to stay in the hospital for a week, after which I was fitted with a draconian brace that I had to wear for three months. The doctor told me that my prognosis was good, but that most likely, by the age of 40, I would experience recurring back pain.

I was 12 years old at the time, so "by the age of 40" didn't have much meaning for me. But now, almost thirty-five years later at the age of 46, I can tell you the doctor was right. For the last few years, when it gets cold and damp outside, my back has really ached.

Mine is not the typical back problem, but I'm by no means alone when it comes to pain and its debilitating effects. After the common cold, back problems are the most frequent cause of missed workdays in adults under 45. Women, while nursing and carrying their babies around all day, often feel crimps in their backs and necks. And 60 to 90 percent of *all* adults suffer back pain at some point in their lives. Indeed, back pain, lower back pain in particular, ranks fifth among the most frequent reasons for hospitalizations.

In dollar terms, the U.S. spends anywhere from $30 to $70 billion each year on medical care to relieve back pain. That's more than twice as much as is spent on all care for cancer patients.

The good news: Most back pain is not caused by a serious injury like the one I had. It's usually the result of short-term stress on the muscles and ligaments that support the spine, coming from daily activities like bending, lifting heavy objects the wrong way, and sitting too long. (It's thought that back pain has been on the rise in recent decades because most people now sit much longer than they ever did.)

The even better news: Simple lifestyle measures can do much to ameliorate back pain—and even prevent it altogether. I have seen this over and over again in my role as director of the John Hancock Center for Physical Activity and Nutrition at Tufts, and in research reported by others in the field as well.

I practice those measures pretty regularly, which allows me to be in less pain, much less often, than I otherwise would be. Imagine what they would do for someone with back pain resulting from minor aches and strains rather than the trauma I put my own back through.

The lifestyle measures I'm talking about are not what most people think, which is why, as someone who knows back pain first-hand, I have decided to write this book.

It is often assumed that the best way to take care of a bad back is always to rest it. In fact, even until recently, back patients were routinely sent to bed for weeks or even months. But in just about all cases, taking it too easy can actually make the pain worse. That's because remaining sedentary for too long can result in stiff, weakened back muscles and less elastic ligaments that make sitting, standing, bending, and general moving around even *more* difficult. Indeed, a sedentary lifestyle is a strong *predictor* of back pain.

Movement, on the other hand (which should be resumed in most cases just twenty-four to forty-eight hours after back pain begins), is nourishing to the spine. It pumps fluid into the discs that cushion the vertebrae, keeping them at peak sponginess and therefore best able to act as shock absorbers. Then, too, movement increases the strength and flexibility of all the muscles in the trunk—including those in the abdomen as well as in the back. That's important because the spine is like scaffolding that depends on support from all sides, not just from behind.

Molly, a woman who once wrote to me, knows this firsthand. She had injured her back ten years earlier and just assumed the pain would go away. But it didn't. Over the course of a year, she stopped exercising entirely. In fact, she said, "I became afraid of exercise."

One day, her husband wanted to teach her how to cross-country ski. "I was so nervous about my back," she wrote, "that I was shaking." But Molly went, anyway. "And when I got home," she reported, "I found that my back felt so much better. It was a lightbulb going off; strength begets strength."

While it took Molly ten years to get over her fear that exercising would make her back pain worse—and to realize that exercise *blunted* back pain—you will be spared the long wait, and all the years of fear and seeming disability, by virtue of reading this book and following through with its recommendations. For instance, you'll be shown exercises that *directly* target the back.

The best kinds of movement: strength-training exercises combined with stretching (flexibility moves) and a moderate amount of aerobic activity. The latest research shows quite clearly that progressive strength training decreases pain in people with chronic back discomfort, which makes sense since the back muscles of sedentary individuals are very weak and cannot support the back the way they should.

Chapter 4 will equip you with exactly the exercise program your back needs. It's tailored specifically for women—not so taxing that you might risk further injury, but just challenging enough that you will strengthen the back components that will keep you from further pain—and prevent back pain in the future.

There's more to lifestyle than exercise for supporting your back, however. It is now well known that stress and depression heighten pain, including back pain, so relaxation techniques ease pressure on the back as well. They include massage, tai chi, meditation, yoga, psy-

Stronger Back, Trimmer Tummy

As I pass through my mid-40s, I can relate to the concern over a thickening middle, which a lot of women ask me about. They're not happy that their tummies used to look pretty flat and have now expanded. For better or worse, as women grow older, gains in abdominal thickness are typical.

Unfortunately, it's not just aesthetically unappealing. It also has health consequences. A thick midsection puts you at increased risk for chronic conditions such as heart disease and diabetes. It puts undue strain on your back as well.

The good news is that regular exercise really *can* stem the tide of an expanding middle. Several of our exercise studies at Tufts University, in fact, have shown losses of body fat and inches off the waist.

How, exactly, do you do it? Strength training, combined with aerobic exercise (the program in this book), is the key. Strength training the back (and abdominal) muscles helps improve your posture and thereby minimizes the slouch that can make your tummy stick out. But a casing of fat surrounds those muscles. And you need aerobic activities to minimize the gain in body fat over the years and to *burn* off excess fat that may already be sitting there. You may not get back the exact figure you had at 20, but an ever-expanding midsection is by no means inevitable. You can look fit and fine at 40, 50, 60, and beyond.

chotherapy, Alexander Technique, and even just reaching out to others. All of these will be discussed in chapter 5.

Ergonomics, the relation of your body to its environment, is also very important to back support, which is why chapter 6 will give specifics on how to make your work and home spaces environmentally correct. Did you know that if you work at a computer, there's a certain number of inches that should separate your face from the monitor so as not to put undue pressure on your spine? Or that crooking the phone under your shoulder as you multitask with papers is really bad for your neck and back muscles, and that there's a simple solution for those who want to talk on the phone and do something else at the same time? How you organize your kitchen and what kind of mattress you sleep on—and how often you replace it—also are ergonomic points that have to be taken into consideration if you're going to be as good to your back as possible.

Of course, sometimes lifestyle isn't enough by itself to give an aching back what it needs. You might need to see a health care professional. Your primary care physician is integral to your plan of action, but there are specialists who might be able to help you as well: a chiropractor, an acupuncturist, or a physical therapist, for instance.

Some people automatically assume chiropractors and acupuncturists are quacks, but most are legitimate practitioners who really can help you. You just have to know what to expect from them. You also have to know their limitations, as with any other health care provider, as well as how to choose one who is properly credentialed. Chapter 7 will cue you to all the ins and outs for choosing a good health care provider in addition to your primary care physician, in case your back needs some extra help from the outside.

What if, in the end, all your efforts to ease back pain via lifestyle and perhaps various health care professionals don't provide relief? Should you then consider back surgery? It's a very reasonable question for someone in chronic pain, but with a somewhat complicated answer. There's a lot you need to know before deciding to go under the knife (or laser beam!). Chapter 8 will give you the specifics so that you can participate in making an informed decision. You *have to* participate. Surgery for back pain is almost always elective. The doctor, in the end, will leave the choice up to you.

To make such a choice, and, in fact, to make all decisions concerning the care of your back, you need to understand exactly what the back is made of and how it works. Knowledge in this case really is empowerment. That's why, before I get to strategizing with you on how to reduce your pain and prevent discomfort down the line, I will explain in chapter 2 just what the back is composed of and how the different elements work together. Did you know, for instance, that the spine is actually an S-shaped curve of vertebrae, or bones, reaching from the base of the skull to the top of the pelvis? Or that the five lowest vertebrae in this chain of bones—the lumbar spine—are where most people experience back pain? And were you aware that spongy discs between each vertebra act like back joints, keeping the bones from rubbing against each other? And that slouching or a potbelly will pull the spine forward and make those "joints" more vulnerable to injury? The information will give you mental images of how your back works, which in turn will provide motivation for you to take the steps necessary to keep your back in the best shape possible.

You'll also be given information, in chapter 3, on the most common causes of back pain, which include everyday mishaps such as lifting improperly and using poor posture.

With this knowledge in hand, the approaches I outline will work. Yes, I had serious trauma to my back, but I can still live a full and active life that's largely free of back pain. Most women, whose back injuries never land them in the hospital, can certainly become free of most, if not all, of the back pain that may plague them. Women in my research studies have confirmed this to me time and time again.

Taking care of your back health is *literally* at the core of your being. While it would be wonderful to hear that one simple exercise can make the difference, the truth is more complicated than that. The strategy that incorporates a focus on the body, the mind, *and* your environment will have the most effective and longest lasting outcome.

Here's to your own strong and healthy back. I know you have what it takes to get you there.

Understanding Your Back: Anatomy and Physiology

◈

fter the brain, the trunk is the most complex part of the body. It's not just because it contains our vital organs—the heart, kidneys, lungs, stomach, liver, intestines, sex organs, and so on. It's also that the architecture of the trunk is so much more intricate than that of the arms or legs. Each limb has just a few bones and muscles. But the trunk has many, which makes sense when you consider that the spine inside it needs to be able to flex, extend, and twist more than almost any other part of the body. Think about bending sideways to pick up a pencil, or reaching for something on a high shelf, or "folding yourself in" a little to cradle a baby. The spine in the center of the trunk is "Movement Central," capable of initiating bodily motion in more ways than you may realize.

SPINAL OVERVIEW

Running right down the center of the back is the spinal column, which contains many of the trunk's bones, called vertebrae. It also contains the spinal cord, which houses the nerves of the central nervous system. The trunk has ligaments, too. They form a casing of sorts around the vertebrae.

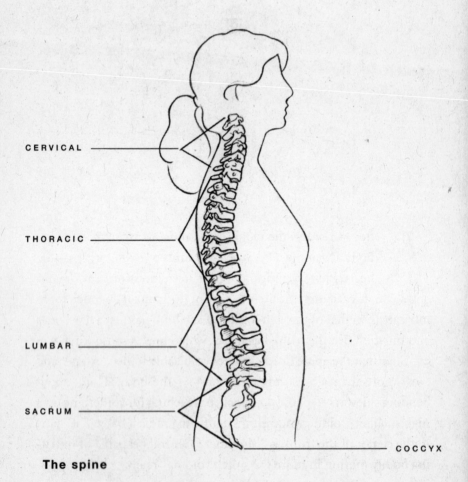

CERVICAL

THORACIC

LUMBAR

SACRUM

COCCYX

The spine

The Vertebrae

No doubt you've seen illustrations of the vertebrae, the series of bones in the back that are stacked on top of each other in such a way as to form an S if you look from the side. That S, or vertebral column, gives your body shape and definition. Without it you'd be a puddle.

The vertebral column starts at the base of the skull and extends to the tailbone, consisting of four regions that contain roughly thirty bones. The cervical region supports the head and neck and has seven vertebrae. The thoracic region—essentially the middle of the back—contains twelve vertebrae. The lower back is composed of the lumbar region, or lumbar spine, with five vertebrae. (These are the largest vertebrae of all and the ones that are usually measured during a bone density test.) The lowest part of the vertebral column consists of the sacrum and coccyx, or tailbone. When we are children, the sacrum is made up of five separate vertebrae, and the coccyx, of four. But by the time we reach adulthood, those bones have fused, leaving just one bone for the sacrum and one for the coccyx. The sacrum is attached to the pelvis via what is called the sacroiliac joint. This particular joint has little movement or flexibility due to strong ligaments that keep it stable.

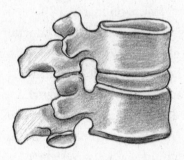

Vertebrae

Vertebrae other than the sacrum and coccyx do allow for flexibility. Every time two bones come together, they form a joint that makes it possible to twist, tuck, and extend—sideways, forward, and backward.

The way the vertebrae come together is unlike the way bones come together anywhere else in the body. The "body" of each vertebra, made of spongy, porous bone, is cylindrical. Coming out of the back end of the vertebral body are pieces of bone called pedicles, which in turn attach to the processes (spinal and transverse). These are bony protuberances. You can feel the processes if you run your hand down someone's back. They're the little bumps that run much of the back's length.

But there's much more to the processes than you can feel. They flare to the right and left and also up and down, achieving two basic functions. One is to connect each vertebra to the next; the processes interlock something like complicated Lego pieces to allow the vertebrae to fit snugly, one on top of the other. That allows enough give for flexible movement but not so much that a good twist would allow the whole apparatus to fall apart. The processes' other function, as they branch outward from the pedicles that attach them to the vertebral bodies, is to form a cavity, or protective cage, for the spinal cord, which contains much of the central nervous system necessary for all feeling and movement. (More on that in a bit.)

Between the vertebrae are discs, which function much the way that cartilage does in all the other joints of the body. They take up the space between two bones—the joint—and, when in good shape, keep bones from scraping against each other and causing pain during movement. Each disc is made of a tough, fibrous casing that surrounds a gelatinous inside. That combination of materials is what provides crucial cushioning between vertebrae. If a disc ruptures, the jellylike center can ooze out into surrounding tissues, irritating nerves and causing pain. If enough compression occurs, the disc becomes so flat that you get bone on bone as you move about—a very painful predicament.

Other Back Bones

The thirty or so bones that form the vertebral column are not the only bones in the trunk. There are also the ribs, pelvis, collarbones, and scapulae. The ribs, a bony cage formed by twelve pairs of bones that protect the heart and lungs, all come out of the thoracic vertebrae. The top seven of the rib pairs, called true ribs, connect in the front of the body to the sternum, a piece of cartilage between the breasts. The sternum helps the ribs remain suspended sort of like a wire basket; that keeps them fixed but with some give. The next two to three rib pairs do not connect to the sternum. Rather, they connect to the ribs above them with the help of cartilage. The lowest two rib pairs just "float." They are not connected in the front of the body at all.

You're Taller in the Morning

Each of the back's discs, cylindrical in shape, is about one quarter to three quarters of an inch thick. Overnight, while you are sleeping, the discs absorb water and become a little thicker, making you taller. By the end of the day, gravity has done its work, and the excess fluid has been squeezed out of the discs, making you a half inch or so shorter again. If you measure your height periodically—which you should as a crude indication of whether you may have osteoporosis or other back problems—make sure to always do it at the same time in the morning to get your true height.

The pelvis, made up of two bones that connect at both the front and the back, holds the reproductive system—the uterus and ovaries—as well as the digestive system, which allows the nutrients in our food to be absorbed by our bodies and the waste to be eliminated. Shaped like a saddle, the pelvis is also what gives shape to our hips.

The collarbones, along with the scapulae, or shoulder blades (flat, triangular-shaped bones in the upper back), help form the shape and mobility of the shoulders.

The Spinal Cord

Bones allow for movement, but the brain and spinal cord (with all its nerves) are what actually start the process. The brain and spinal nerves "inform" the muscles that are attached to the bones to relax and contract so that movement can take place. (The muscles and bones work in combination with each other to allow for stretching, reaching, bending, and the like.)

The spinal cord, bathed in spinal fluid, makes its way down the back by threading itself through the processes of the vertebrae. But it also branches out from the vertebral column in many spots along the way, sending pairs of nerves to different areas of the body (right and left) to activate muscles outside of the trunk.

That's why something like numbness in your hands or arms can originate from your neck or back. A nerve to a limb that begins in the spinal column can be pinched between two vertebrae.

Nerves are what sense pain in the body, in fact. They are the grand message system the brain uses, both to mobilize the body and to "hear" if anything is amiss. There are nerves in the central nervous system, which includes the spinal cord, and the peripheral nervous system—thirty-one pairs of nerves that branch out from the spinal cord to the rest of the body.

From the cervical and thoracic regions of the spine, pairs of nerves branch out to control the arms. From the lumbar and sacral regions, nerves branch out to get the hips and legs moving. Nerves branch out from various sections of the spinal cord to keep organs "moving," too. There are nerves for the heart, stomach, uterus, bladder, bowels, etc. All require the nervous system in order to function properly.

The Ligaments

There are three major ligaments in the spinal column. Composed of a tough, fibrous material, they help bones remain attached to other bones as well as to cartilage. The anterior longitudinal ligament runs in front of the vertebral column. The posterior longitudinal ligament runs behind the vertebral column. The third ligament, the *ligamentum flavum,* fills up the openings between vertebrae at the back side of the vertebral column. It helps protect the spinal cord.

Ligaments are extremely important to flexibility. Think of circus contortionists, or even people who can touch their palms to the floor without bending their knees. It's the elasticity of their ligaments (and muscles) that allows for such movements. Some of the elasticity is genetic, but you can improve it with an exercise program, too. The more you improve it, the less likely injuries are to occur, because the back can glide through motions that it wouldn't be able to otherwise.

All Encased by Muscle

If you could peel back your skin and the fat just underneath it, you wouldn't see any vertebrae or other bones. You wouldn't see the

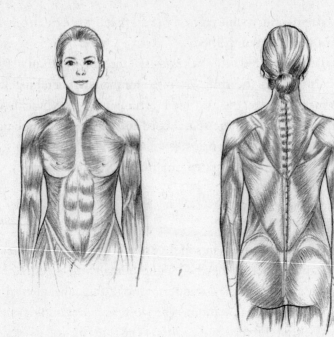

spinal cord, or any ligaments, either. All you'd see are muscles. If the bones support the body, the muscles in the trunk support the bones. They are attached to the bones via tendons, and with instructions from the nerves in the spinal cord, the muscles and bones work in tandem to allow for movement throughout the entire body. Together they create the scaffolding for the trunk—necessary not just for turning, twisting, and bending but also for breathing, giving birth, and a host of other functions. The muscles are so important, in fact, that when you strengthen your back to relieve or ward off pain, it's largely the muscles that you're directly working on.

The Back Is Also the Front

When people think of the back, they think of that part between the neck and the buttocks that they can't see. But the whole trunk is involved in back health, including your abdominal muscles, because *the back needs support from all sides.* When you strengthen your abdominals through exercise, you're relieving pressure on the spine because you're shifting some of the burden of movement and posture away from it.

That allows the spine to be more flexible, easing up areas where nerves come out. The end result is that the nerves are much less likely to become pinched and cause pain in the back—or other areas of the body.

Such will be the case for you when you strengthen your back—and front—with the strength training exercises recommended in chapter 4. And the increased flexibility in your muscles, ligaments, and tendons that comes from the stretching exercises advised in that chapter will give you more elasticity, reducing the risk for injury when you move your back—and even when you're just sitting still or moving gently in your seat.

CHAPTER 3

The Major Causes of Back Pain

◆

The discs in my lumbar spine started degenerating by the time I was in my 20s—I inherited the tendency from my parents. At one point the pain in my lower back got so bad after I bent over to pick up my toddler that I couldn't stand up straight for several days.

—Anne

Ten percent of people in the United States can expect some back pain during any given year, and as many as four in five people will experience pain in their backs over the course of their lives. Often, it is relatively mild and resolves within a couple of months. But one in four Americans suffers from back pain chronically.

The most common area of back pain is the lumbar region—the lower back. In fact, low back pain is the second most common complaint that drives people into doctors' offices.

THE LOWER BACK WORKS HARDEST

The reason most back pain occurs in the lower region is that the lumbar section—that curve in the spine—is more responsible for the body's weight load than the upper back. The lower back also takes the lion's share of the burden for twisting, turning, and lifting—all movements that occur much more frequently than may be readily apparent.

Stand up for a minute and twist from side to side. For many people, it all happens near the hips rather than the shoulders. Now think about how often you twist or bend—to reach for something, to turn toward someone, to pick something up, and so on. That's a lot of repeated insult to the lower back. Granted, the vertebrae in the lumbar region are larger than elsewhere in the back to afford extra protection, but all that movement every day still takes its toll. Compounding the problem is that the lower back muscles are often out of shape, making them all the less likely to be up to the task of supporting all the upper body's movements and all the more likely to end up sprained, pulled, or otherwise injured.

DECONDITIONING LEAVES THE BACK WIDE OPEN TO PAIN

Anywhere in the body that you have strong muscles, you're less prone to pain, injury, and fatigue. Condition your hip, thigh, and calf muscles by walking every day, and your legs won't tire so easily. Lift weights regularly, and you'll be able to carry more. Exercise the muscles in your back, and your back will be less likely to give you problems.

Since the back, particularly the lower back, is used so often, you'd think it was one area of the body that gets a lot of physical activity without your making a conscious effort to exercise the muscles there. But ironically, even many of the fittest people you see around you—people who engage in aerobic exercises like jogging and who strength train regularly—have weak back muscles. The muscles tend to be left both weak and inflexible due to a lack of conditioning.

If we were all stone masons, rigorously exercising those muscles every day in the course of our work, they'd be strong. But most people in modern society, even athletic people, sit for a good part of the day and are rather sedentary. They don't generally *need* their lower backs for heavy work. Thus, in a rare moment when the lower back gets called into play for a heavy-duty move, or when the accumulated smaller insults to the lumbar region cross a certain line, the back is not up to the challenge. The result of putting more pressure on the lumbar spine than it's used to taking: pain. (Those who sit behind a desk all day are particularly prone to back pain.)

The back pain can be acute, lasting less than two weeks; subacute, lasting up to twelve weeks; or chronic, lasting longer than twelve weeks. It can be dull or excruciatingly sharp.

BEYOND DECONDITIONING

Deconditioning of the back muscles is the overarching reason for the epidemic of back pain in the United States. But there are many other problems that dovetail with general back weakness and inflexibility, making pain that much more likely.

- *Excess body weight.* It stands to reason that since the lower back supports so much of the body's weight, the more extra

pounds someone carries, the greater the strain on the lumbar spine with every turn and bend.

- *Smoking.* It's unclear exactly why smoking continues to come
up as a risk factor for back problems. But it does. Smokers
also have a poorer prognosis in the event of a back injury, especially one that requires surgery.
- *Poor posture.* Chronic poor posture—a habitual tendency to
slump forward—can force the bones in the spine out of alignment. That creates pressure on the nerves, which are literal
pain sensors.
- *Poor muscle flexibility.* Numerous studies have linked back
pain to a lack of flexibility. For example, tight hamstring muscles (at the back of the thighs) have a strong association with
low back pain—and the greatest impact on range of motion.
Relatively inflexible hip flexor muscles also tend to go hand
in hand with lower back pain.

STRUCTURAL CAUSES OF BACK PAIN

Aside from the psychological factors, the causes of back pain described above are directly in your control. Keep your back muscles in
shape, maintain or reach a healthy body weight, don't smoke, stand
up and sit straight, and work toward keeping your muscles flexible,
and your back will be much less prone to pain—and will recover
more quickly should you experience pain.

But there are many things you don't make happen but that happen *to you,* that can affect your chances of having bouts of back pain.
Technically, these causes of back pain are called nonmodifiable,
which makes it sound as though you're stuck with the discomfort.
But you're not—at least not entirely. Keep in mind as you read

Is It All in Your Head?

Some people go from doctor to doctor, trying to find the cause of their back pain, only ending up distrustful of the medical community because doctors can't find anything wrong and insist, one after another, that it's all in the patient's head. The thing is, back pain may very well originate in some people's heads. But that doesn't make it any less real.

In some people, for reasons not yet understood, depression leads to back pain. In others, lack of sleep can induce back discomfort. In still others, stress can be the back pain trigger, which makes intuitive sense. Stress leads to muscle tension, and if the muscles in the back, particularly the upper back and neck, are constantly tensed, they can spasm and cause considerable discomfort. Making matters worse still, depression in the face of stress can affect the way a person handles her back problem, leading to a slower recovery.

Both depression and stress are eminently treatable by the medical community. Great strides have been made, both via therapy and pharmacology, in treating those conditions, which in turn can remove psychological stumbling blocks to treating pain. There are also a number of nonmedical approaches, such as massage, that can reduce emotional tension, as chapter 5 will make clear.

But what has also come to light is that regular exercise, without professional intervention, can help alleviate both depression and stress. It may be the sense of empowerment born of making the body stronger that helps mitigate negative emotional states. Or perhaps it's just the structure and discipline of an exercise program that helps— the sense of getting control over one's life. Exercise elevates brain endorphin levels, too. Whatever the reason, the same exercise that can condition a weak back can also help dispel psychological contributors to back pain.

through these causes that there is, in fact, much you can do both to prevent and ameliorate the brunt of pain that ensues from structural causes, as I will explain shortly.

- *Degenerative discs.* With age, the discs connecting the bones in the spine begin to deteriorate and flatten. That makes for less cushioning between the vertebrae. Not all older people experience back pain as a result, but it does increase their chances.
- *Scoliosis.* Scoliosis, or curvature of the spine, creates an imbalance (you can actually see that the spine is not straight when you look at it), so that the shoulder and hip on one side of the body are a little higher than the other. In some cases, when a genetic abnormality causes the legs to be slightly different lengths, scoliosis develops as a child's spine grows on an uneven base.
- *Compression fractures due to osteoporosis.* One in four women over 60 experiences at least one wedge or crush fracture in the spine as a result of osteoporosis, the degenerative bone disease. Typically, such fractures cause either kyphosis (a hump on the upper part of the back sometimes referred to as a dowager's hump) or lordosis (in which the lower back bows forward and pushes out the stomach, which results in sort of a potbelly). Either way, the curvature of the spine can cause muscle strain, nerve damage, and pain.
- *Trauma or sports injuries.* Fractured vertebrae or other parts of the spine result not just from osteoporosis but also from accidents such as falls, car wrecks, and sports injuries, like the one I had as a child.
- *Herniated disc.* Also called a slipped disc, this condition results when a disc has ruptured, usually from strenuous phys-

ical activity, such as lifting something too heavy. The disc then spills its jellylike contents into the spinal column, irritating nerves there and causing pain.

• *Arthritis.* The most common type of arthritis is osteoarthritis, which can cause bone spurs—small bony outgrowths that may prove very painful. In the back, arthritis-related bone spurs tend to occur in the facet joints. That's where the processes (discussed in chapter 2) join together in the back of the vertebrae.

  Rheumatoid arthritis can result in back pain, too, although that is less common. The pain, caused by inflammation between vertebrae, tends to occur in the upper back.

• *Paget's disease.* A rare condition, Paget's disease causes bone to break down abnormally and then re-form at a greater rate, creating *excessive* bone. The resulting pain in the back can be extreme.

• *Spinal stenosis.* Also called spinal narrowing, spinal stenosis occurs when ligaments thicken at the spinal column, through which the spinal cord runs. That narrowing puts pressure on the cord, which causes pain. There can even be significant numbness and tingling in the legs, sometimes coupled with constipation or bowel or urinary incontinence.

WHEN THE CAUSE OF THE PAIN ISN'T STRUCTURAL

The various reasons for back pain discussed above are all structural, by which I mean there's a mechanical, or anatomical, abnormality in the back that's causing the problem. But there are some reasons for back pain that are nonstructural yet are also not related to lifestyle; the source of the discomfort stems from something else entirely. These causes of back pain require medical attention that in some cases don't even have anything to do with the back:

- *Infections.* Urinary tract infections can bring on referred pain to the lower back. A bone infection called osteomyelitis, usually caused by bacteria, can also create back pain. The infection often starts in bone tissue in another part of the body and then spreads to the back via the blood.
- *Cancer.* Leukemia, lymphoma, and multiple myeloma all can lead to back pain, as can bone cancer and other malignancies that make their way into the spinal cord.
- *Conditions of the pelvic organs.* Endometriosis, in which uterine cells multiply in areas outside the uterus (such as on the ovaries or fallopian tubes) can in some cases lead to severe back pain, as can chronic pelvic inflammatory disease.
- *Kidney stones.* The kidneys are located in the lower back. Any time they are compromised, back pain can result.
- *Menstruation.* The sloughing of the endometrial lining during menstruation can cause cramping and lower back pain. If it's severe, it could be a sign of endometriosis.

MODIFYING WHAT'S SUPPOSEDLY NOT MODIFIABLE

No matter how fit you are, no matter how trim, any condition on the preceding lists can strike you. And in that sense, all of them are in a

Sciatica Is a *Symptom*

You may have heard people say they're suffering from back pain because of sciatica. And they may be. But sciatica, pain along the large sciatic nerve that runs from the lower back through the buttocks and along the back of each leg, is a symptom of an underlying problem. For example, it can be brought on either by a herniated disc or spinal stenosis. It is not a root cause of back pain.

certain way nonmodifiable. You cannot prevent rheumatoid arthritis, scoliosis, or menstruation.

That said, however, there is much you can do to minimize back pain, and in some cases eliminate it altogether, with proper conditioning and other lifestyle steps. You may even be able to prevent back pain, whether or not the cause is modifiable.

It all goes back to strong, flexible muscles. Take degenerative discs. There might be nothing in your lifestyle choices that could help stop the disc deterioration that leads to pain. But if the muscles around your discs are strong and supple, they can compensate to a large degree for the movements that the discs cannot handle well, taking pressure off and thereby relieving—and even staving off—pain.

It's the same for osteoporosis. The bones in your back may be very prone to fractures, and you may even have already suffered a back fracture. But the back muscles, properly conditioned, can allow the body to "work around" weakened bones to a significant extent.

My own history illustrates the point. When I broke my back more than thirty years ago, my doctor told me that I could expect to have a "bad" back in adult life. He was right. During my first pregnancy, at 27, my back hurt so much that I literally felt as though I wasn't going to make it. And after giving birth to each of my three children, repeatedly bending over to nurse, diaper, and such, continually aggravated the pain. By the time I reached my late 30s, I would have significant pain in the middle of my back for about a month every winter, when the weather was particularly cold and damp. Both at work and at home I would keep a heating pad on my back or lie on the floor to relieve the pain.

Interestingly, while I have been strength-training and participating in all kinds of vigorous activity for years, I had always stayed away from exercises that targeted my middle back. In retrospect, I suppose it's because I was so weak in that area to begin with and the exercises were uncomfortable, to boot. But a rehabilitation doctor finally convinced me that the muscles in my middle back were the very ones I most needed to challenge.

I took a leap of faith and followed her directions to work my mid back muscles through specific exercise routines. I can't say that I no longer ever experience a moment's discomfort in my back. But the pain has subsided to the point that a few years ago I began to engage in a *recreational* activity that requires hard use of the back muscles—rock climbing. The rock climbing has reinforced the effects of the exercises, and vice versa. My back isn't nearly as bad as the doctor from my childhood predicted.

Whether your back pain is due to an injury, deconditioning, or something else, the same can be true for you. That's what the rest of this book is about—helping you overcome, and even prevent, back pain that you may have perhaps come to believe is not modifiable.

You'll have to be consistent in your efforts to get results. You won't be able to expect much if you follow the program in a haphazard manner. But the steps I recommend you take are not difficult; you don't have to become a rock climber. You just have to be willing to prod your body into cooperating with you. If you can commit to giving it just a little more than an hour a week, you'll get much freedom from pain, as well as greater flexibility of movement, in return.

PART 2

The Strong Back Action Plan

CHAPTER 4

The
Strong Women, Strong Backs
Exercise Program

I've had lower back pain all my life, and tingling and numbness since I was in my 20s. I started strength-training in the early nineties, but one of the areas I always avoided was my trunk. I thought that exercising that part of my body would make my spinal symptoms worse. But a physical therapist I started seeing a few years ago said I needed to work through those feelings and just trust on the other end that I would have good results. Now, if I go a few days where I don't strength-train my trunk muscles, I feel stiffer, and the symptoms start coming on more.

—JOSEPHINE

It's one of those instances in which both intuitive and counter-intuitive logic come into play. Intuitively, it makes sense that a back that's strong and flexible is going to be a back that's healthy—and also bounces back from pain as quickly as possible should you end up hurting it. But it may feel counterintuitive to challenge parts of your body that feel uncomfortable.

However you look at it, an exercise program that specifically targets the back is crucial. It strengthens the muscles, meaning your back can take on challenges that would otherwise put it "out"; and it increases back flexibility—your ability to twist and turn and bend as needed without wrenching something out of alignment.

That's what the exercise program in this chapter is about. Designed specifically for women (our backs are more delicate than men's), it outlines the best exercises for increasing strength in your back muscles. In designing the plan, I essentially took the trunk apart to make sure each area of the back and abdomen would be tackled. The program will also improve flexibility along your entire spine, from your neck to your tailbone. It draws upon research that has been published over the years regarding moves that strengthen the back without putting it at risk; consultations with numerous health professionals; and my own personal experience improving strength where I broke my back many years ago.

While strength-training exercises are at the heart of the program, followed closely by stretches that increase flexibility, there is also an aerobic component. Yes, you want to target your back, but you have to get your whole body moving and in shape. The back does not operate in isolation.

Don't be concerned that my recommendations are going to add up to an impossible time commitment. I'm talking about just a few hours a week, spread out over as little as three days. Of course, carving even a few hours a week out of a schedule that's already squeezed to the max might seem impossible. But your back and trunk health are worth it, as is the rest of your body. Reading this book is one thing, but you have to follow through to get the desired results.

Josephine, the woman quoted at the beginning of this chapter, describes it better than I can, and can attest to the benefits to her back as well: "I feel more steady. I'm still skiing and biking. Walking long distances and standing for long periods of time can be painful, but the exercise has definitely kept things moving. It's the most critical factor."

Do not rush the plan I have laid out for you. The best way to incorporate exercise into your life, whether for your back or in general, is to adapt your body to it gradually. Go too quickly, and you'll be more prone to give up before your efforts really get underway. You'll be more prone to injure yourself, too. Go slowly and deliberately, and within just a few weeks you'll start to feel different—younger. Your back will start to improve if it has been weak (imagine the freedom of not holding your hand to the bottom of your back after you've lifted something heavy), and you will feel stronger overall if you had a good back to begin with and want to keep it that way.

BEFORE YOU BEGIN

Before you start the program, I strongly recommend that you take the PAR-Q (Physical Activity Readiness Questionnaire) that follows. I know things like this often seem like a bother—you just want to get going. And the truth is, most women *can* participate in this back exercise program without any concerns that their body can't handle it. But by taking just a couple of minutes' extra time to answer a few questions, you'll be guaranteeing that the plan is safe for you, or, in some cases, deciding to see a doctor before you take up more vigorous physical activity than you may have been used to. (A note to those over 70 and anyone with acute back problems: PAR-Q or not, it's important that you get your doctor's thumbs-up before embarking on this program.)

PAR-Q & YOU

(A Questionnaire for People Aged 15 to 69)

Regular physical activity is fun and healthy, and increasingly more people are starting to become more active every day. Being more active is very safe for most people. However, some people should check with their doctor before they start becoming much more physically active.

If you are planning to become much more physically active than you are now, start by answering the seven questions in the box below. If you are between the ages of 15 and 69, the PAR-Q will tell you if you should check with your doctor before you start. If you are over 69 years of age, and you are not used to being very active, check with your doctor.

Common sense is your best guide when you answer these questions. Please read the questions carefully and answer each one honestly: check YES or NO.

YES	NO	
☐	☐	1. Has your doctor ever said that you have a heart condition <u>and</u> that you should only do physical activity recommended by a doctor?
☐	☐	2. Do you feel pain in your chest when you do physical activity?
☐	☐	3. In the past month, have you had chest pain when you were not doing physical activity?
☐	☐	4. Do you lose your balance because of dizziness or do you ever lose consciousness?
☐	☐	5. Do you have a bone or joint problem that could be made worse by a change in your physical activity?
☐	☐	6. Is your doctor currently prescribing drugs (for example, water pills) for your blood pressure or heart condition?
☐	☐	7. Do you know of <u>any other reason</u> why you should not do physical activity?

IF YOU ANSWERED

YES to one or more questions

Talk with your doctor by phone or in person BEFORE you start becoming much more physically active or BEFORE you have a fitness appraisal. Tell your doctor about the PAR-Q and which questions you answered YES.

+ You may be able to do any activity you want—as long as you start slowly and build up gradually. Or, you may need to restrict your activities to those which are safe for you. Talk with your doctor about the kinds of activities you wish to participate in and follow his/her advice.
+ Find out which community programs are safe and helpful for you.

NO to all questions

If you answered NO honestly to <u>all</u> PAR-Q questions, you can be reasonably sure that you can:

+ start becoming much more physically active—begin slowly and build up gradually. This is the safest and easiest way to go.
+ take part in a fitness appraisal—this is an excellent way to determine your basic fitness so that you can plan the best way for you to live actively.

DELAY BECOMING MUCH MORE ACTIVE:

+ if you are not feeling well because of a temporary illness such as a cold or fever—wait until you feel better; or
+ if you are or may be pregnant—talk to your doctor before you start becoming more active.

Please note: If your health changes so that you then answer YES to any of the above questions, tell your fitness or health professional. Ask whether you should change your physical activity plan.

Appropriate Clothing and Equipment

The program is simple, and you probably have some, but not all, of what you need to get you going. Here's a rundown of essentials required for you to do the exercises correctly and safely. You won't have to shell out too much money.

Athletic Shoes

Do you own a pair of sneakers? How old are they? Did you know that once your athletic shoes are six to nine months old, it's time to start thinking about your next pair? Here's how to determine whether your athletic shoes should be replaced:

Put them on a table or counter at eye level. Check whether the soles are worn, both on the outside and inside edges. If so, it's time to make a trip to the shoe store. Exercising with shoes that are worn out puts unnecessary stress on the joints. (That's true for all your pairs of shoes, not just those in which you exercise.)

Make sure the salespeople really know how to fit you with the right shoes. They not only have to be comfortable but also have to have the right stability for your gait.

Exercise Mat

You don't absolutely have to have an exercise mat, especially if you have wall-to-wall carpeting. But even then, a firm mat makes floor exercises much more comfortable. It's not expensive—about $18—and it's easy to store. You'll appreciate the extra cushioning.

Stability Ball

For several of the advanced exercises, you will need a stability ball—a large inflated rubber ball that you either sit or lean on as you go through the strength-training moves. The ball should be somewhere between 55 centimeters (22 inches) and 65 centimeters (26 inches) in diameter, depending on your height. You will find it at a sporting-goods store, and also at some larger department stores.

Exercise Bands

Exercise bands are large elastic bands that you can use for several exercises targeting specific muscle groups in the middle and upper back. Make sure to buy three different grades of bands: light, medium, and heavy resistance. It will be helpful (although it's not necessary) if the bands come with small handles that can be attached to the ends. You can buy bands at most sporting-goods stores as well as at online sporting-goods stores. Some department stores carry them, too.

Clothing

If you have some loose, nonrestrictive clothing, you have everything you need. You just want to make sure that your tops and bottoms allow you a full range of motion (and keep you warm enough when doing aerobic exercises outdoors in winter—layers work best).

Water

Contrary to popular belief, it is not necessary to drink at least eight glasses of water a day. For most people, thirst is an adequate guide to fluid needs (unless, of course, it is very hot, in which case you should go a little beyond quenching your thirst). Still, I think it's a reasonable precaution to drink some water just before and after an aerobic workout and to have some handy during strength training, too. You most certainly don't need a sports drink for this exercise program, with all of its calories. Sports drinks are for aerobic activities that last for at least one and a half hours *at a time* (or if you are working out for a long time in hot weather).

THE *STRONG WOMEN, STRONG BACKS* EXERCISE PROGRAM

Here is the exercise program at a glance. As I said before, you can realize significant benefits working out as few as three days per week. But of course, over time, in order to reap the greatest gains, you may want to increase the frequency and duration of your exercise sessions.

Strength training:	20 minutes at a time, three to five days a week
Flexibility (stretching):	5–10 minutes following every strength-training session (more often if you desire)
Aerobics:	30 or more minutes at a time, three to six days a week

It may seem like a lot, particularly if you're not used to exercising, or haven't done so for a number of years. But if you're serious about improving your back and making it less prone to pain, this is the commitment you need to make.

As I said earlier, it doesn't have to happen all at once. You'll build the changes into your lifestyle little by little. Before long, rather than seeming onerous, exercise will be something you won't want to go without.

Strength Training

These are the core exercises (no pun intended) for the *Strong Women, Strong Backs* exercise program. Strengthening the muscles of the core, or trunk—those in the back as well as the front—will have the greatest impact on your back health. Specifically, the strength training exercises you'll be doing target muscles in the chest, abdomen, lower back, hips, midback, and upper back and shoulders. In other words, the entire scaffolding of the back will be targeted (see illustration on page 18).

I recommend you do these exercises three to five days a week. *This is an exception to the usual rule of strength training.* Just about all strength-training exercise can safely be performed no more than three days a week because the muscles being exercised need a day off in between exercise sessions. Strength training causes little microtears in muscle, which is good because that's what allows the muscles to increase their capacity. But not allowing the muscles enough time to recover from exercise sessions leaves them more, rather than less, prone to injury.

. The reason these exercises are different is that the intensity required isn't as great as for other strength-training moves, especially at the beginning. That's what makes it safe to do them two days in a row. Every other day will certainly be helpful, but results will come about more slowly than if you do them five days a week.

There are five strength-training exercises in the routine, with a sixth one added once you gain a certain amount of strength. All of them not only will make your back muscles stronger, they will also improve stability.

Each time you do one of the exercises—whether it's lifting your arms out to your sides or raising your chest off the floor while lying down—you have completed a repetition, or rep. Ten reps make a set, and for most exercises, you want to complete *two sets of each exercise per exercise session.* You should always rest for a minute or so between sets.

Figuring Out the Right Strength Training Intensity

If you can easily perform more than 10 reps in a row, you're not sufficiently challenging your muscles. And if you can only complete

5 or 6 reps in good form before you have to stop, you're pushing your muscles too hard. Here's how to gauge whether you're strength-training at the right intensity, which should range from 3 to 4 on the intensity scale. The reps should feel moderately difficult at the start, but well within your capability. By the sixth or seventh rep, the exercise should be noticeably harder. By the time you reach the tenth rep, which you should still be able to do in good form, you should feel like if you didn't stop and wait a little, you couldn't perform another one.

EXERCISE INTENSITY SCALE FOR STRENGTH TRAINING	
EXERCISE INTENSITY LEVEL	**DESCRIPTION OF EFFORT**
1	Very easy: too easy to be noticed, like lifting a pencil.
2	Easy: can be felt but isn't fatiguing, like carrying a book.
3	Moderate: fatiguing only if prolonged—like carrying a full handbag that seems heavier as the day goes on.
4	Hard: more than moderate at first, and becoming difficult by the time you complete six or seven repetitions. You can make the effort 10 times in good form, but need to rest afterward.
5	Extremely hard: requires all your strength, like lifting a piece of heavy furniture that you can only lift once, if at all.

To help you evaluate the intensity of your efforts, I have developed a scale. Use it to determine your intensity at the end of two sets of 10 reps each.

Don't Rush It

You want to get to a point where you're performing each exercise at an intensity of 3 to 4. But when a strength-training exercise is new to you, you should keep the intensity to a 3—or less. That's because the first step is to perfect your form and allow your muscles to become acclimated to a new set of moves. Once you've done the exercise on a few different days, you can go ahead and try to reach an intensity of 3 to 4.

Going from a lesser to a greater intensity means working through what are known as progressions. Just about all of the strength-training moves I recommend here will list various progressions. Always start with the first progression, no matter how easy the exercise might seem to you. Once you master the form, feel free to work up to more difficult progressions.

Ideally, you'll be trying to increase progressions on the order of once a month. But over time, the intervals at which you go from one progression to the next will become more wide-spaced. Remember, no matter what progression you happen to be at, always perform two sets of 10 repetitions. *That* never changes.

After the first few times that you work out, your muscles may feel a little sore. Don't be concerned. That's a signal to you that you are challenging your muscles appropriately. But if the soreness interferes with your routine activities, you're overdoing it. Move down one progression for a few sessions, and then work up again once your muscles have recovered.

Don't feel disheartened if you move through some progressions more slowly than others. Most people begin an exercise program with some muscles stronger than the others, so a little unevenness is bound to occur. Just keep reminding yourself that all of your muscle groups will become stronger if you're consistent in your efforts.

Before You Do the Moves

The safest way to strength train is to *warm up first*. It takes only three to five minutes. Take a brisk walk around the block or even march or dance in place. Just do something before you actually start your strength-training moves.

Timing and Form

You absolutely should not rush through the exercises. The timing of each rep is critical to your doing the exercises properly, and that timing is slower than may feel natural. But remember, you want to ensure that it's your muscles that are doing the work, not gravity and not simple momentum.

For most exercises, one repetition should take about eight seconds altogether. The first three seconds are to actually contract the muscle. Then there's usually a one-second pause, followed by two to three more seconds to allow you to return to the starting position. There is also a pause for you to take a breath before starting the next rep.

After you finish a set of 10 reps, rest for thirty seconds to a minute before going on to the second set. You're not wasting time by doing so. You're allowing blood flow to increase—and thereby allowing nutrients to reach the muscles and metabolic waste to flow away.

The best way to make sure you're doing each exercise in proper form, and thus targeting, or isolating, the appropriate muscles, is to *visualize* the muscles contracting while you lift. Likewise, imagine them lengthening as you return to the starting position. To allow the visualization to work as well as possible, do *not* tense up the other muscles in your body as you're contracting the ones you need to do the rep. Use the brief pause after lifting to scan your body for tension in areas other than the muscles you mean to use. Then purposefully relax those areas. There are a couple of tension hot spots during exercise:

Face: Make sure not to furrow or knit your brow. Also, don't clench your teeth. Keep your jaw loose.

Posture: Keep your shoulders relaxed and your chin in a neutral position. And keep your abdominal muscles firm with your back straight. That doesn't mean to arch your back. It should be relaxed.

Don't Forget to Breathe!

You are never supposed to hold your breath while strength-training, even though it might feel natural to do so at points. Keep breathing throughout. If you don't, you can raise your blood pressure as you lift.

It is best to exhale as you lift (contracting your muscles) and inhale as you return to the starting position (relaxing your muscles). Think of each breath as the energy you need to do the movement. Don't be concerned if you can't get the rhythm going at first. Often, the most difficult part is just remembering to breathe, so just keep on breathing. As you become more comfortable with strength training, the proper breathing rhythm will follow.

I've found, especially for beginners, that it really helps to count *out loud* the seconds during each repetition. This works on two fronts, both allowing you to breathe properly and helping you to do the exercises at the appropriately deliberate tempo.

Strength Training Your Back

The following six exercises were designated for the strength-training component of the *Strong Women, Strong Backs* exercise program because, combined, they will have the greatest impact on your back muscles.

EXERCISE 1: ABDOMINALS ◆

Most people's abdominal muscles, especially women's, are
notoriously weak. And you cannot have a strong back if you
don't have strong abdominals (a strong front) to support
your spine.

Progression 1: Tight Tummy (Basic)

Starting position: Lie flat on the floor with your knees bent and
the soles of your feet on the floor. Place your hands over your lower
stomach.

1-2-Down: Contract your abdominal muscles, which will push
the small of your back toward the floor. You should feel your
tummy get "tight" while you do this. Imagine pulling your belly
button down into the floor.

Hold the move for three seconds.

1-2-Up: Relax and bring yourself back to the starting position.

Reps and sets: Repeat the move 10 times. Rest for thirty seconds
to a minute and then do a second set.

Progression 1

Progression 2

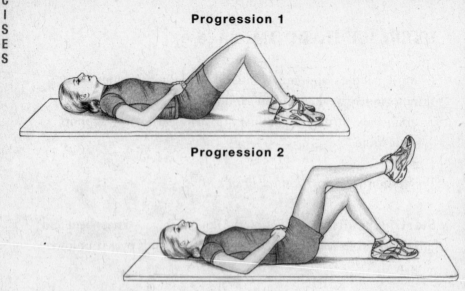

Focal points: Concentrate on breathing throughout this move. If it has been a long time since you have truly felt your abdominal muscles, it will take you some time to really feel that they are working. In these abdominal exercises, the "hold" is where you will feel your muscles working.

Progression 2: Tight Tummy (Intermediate)
The position and the move is the exact same as Tight Tummy (basic), but with the following variation: You raise the lower right leg and hold for three seconds; then while still doing the Tight Tummy, place that leg down and do the same with the left leg, also holding for three seconds. Each repetition takes ten to twelve seconds.

Progression 3: Reverse Curl
The Reverse Curl is a variation on the "crunch." Do not attempt it until you have mastered the other Tight Tummy abdominal moves in good form and they have become easier to do.

Starting position: Sit on the floor with your knees bent and the soles of your feet on the floor. Extend your arms out straight, next to your knees.

1-2-Down: Contract your abdominal muscles, which will push the small of your back toward the floor. You should feel your tummy "get thin" and tight while you do this.

Hold the move for three seconds.

1-2-Up: Relax and bring yourself back to the starting position.

Progression 3

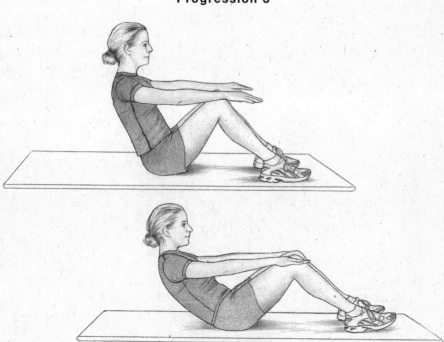

Reps and sets: Repeat the move 10 times. Rest for thirty seconds to a minute and then do the second set.

Focal points: Concentrate on breathing throughout this move. If it has been a long time since you have truly felt your abdominal muscles, it will take you some time to really feel that they are working. Your back should stay in the same position as you contract your abdominal muscles. Remember, the "hold" is where you will feel your muscles working.

EXERCISE 2: CHEST MUSCLES ◆

The muscles underneath the breasts are generally weak to start with. The exercises below will target the upper chest to finish off the front of the trunk.

Progression 1: Counter Push-ups

Starting position: Stand facing a counter (or use a wall) with your feet hip-width apart, knees slightly bent. At arm's length, lightly hold on to the counter (or stand with your palms against the wall).

1-2-3-Forward: Holding your body in a straight line, bend at the elbow to lean your body toward the counter until your head is over the counter edge. You should be at about a 30-degree angle from the starting position.

Pause for a moment.

1-2-Back: Holding your body in a straight line, push with your arms to return to the starting position.

Reps and sets: Complete 10 repetitions. Rest for thirty seconds to a minute and do a second set.

Progression 1

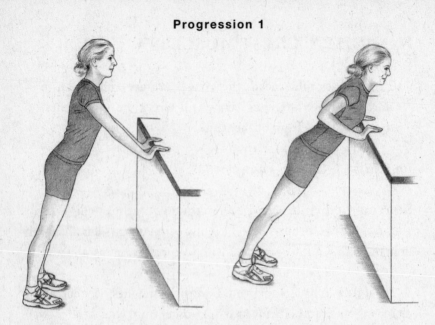

Focal points: Adjust the distance from you to the counter to make it comfortable. If the exercise is too difficult at arm's length, stand closer to the counter/wall. Hold your abdominals tight and shoulders broad to help keep your body straight as you do the exercise.

Progression 2: Modified Push-up
You may not have done push-ups since you were in gym class some decades ago. I promise they are not as bad as you remember! They are also an excellent exercise that targets many important muscle groups in one move. We'll start with a variation that makes the push-up easier to do.

Starting position: Lie flat on your tummy with your palms down, directly next to your shoulders (elbows bent). For increased comfort, use an exercise mat or place a folded towel under your knees.

1-2-Up: Keeping your knees on the floor, push only your chest up in a slow motion. Keep your trunk in a straight line from your head to your knees. Push up until your shoulders are over your hands, but do not lock your elbows.

Pause for a moment.

1-2-3-Down: Slowly lower your torso until your nose is about 4 inches from the floor, keeping your trunk in a straight line.

Reps and sets: Complete 10 repetitions. Rest for thirty seconds to a minute and do a second set.

Progression 2

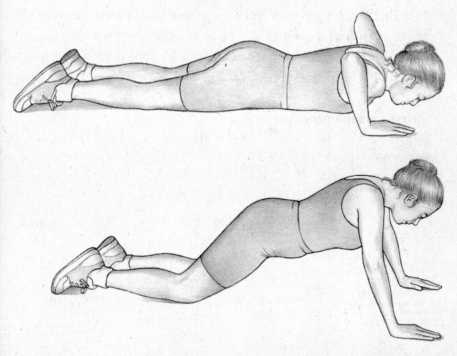

Focal points: Avoid "rolling" yourself up and down. Imagine that your body is a straight line from your head to your knees.

Progression 3: Traditional Push-up

You may have thought that you would never do a "real" push-up. But if you have reached progression 2 with the chest exercises and they have become easy, it is time to move up. You may be able to do only one or two traditional push-ups, but that is great! Do a couple, then go back and finish off the repetitions and sets with the modified version.

Starting position: Lie flat on your tummy with your palms down, directly next to your shoulders (elbows bent). Roll your toes under so that they are on the floor.

1-2-Up: Slowly push your entire body up, supported by your arms and toes. Push all the way up until your shoulders are over your hands, but do not lock your elbows. Your body should be in a straight line from head to heel.

Pause for a moment.

1-2-3-Down: Slowly lower your body until your nose is about 4 inches from the floor, keeping your whole body in a straight line.

Reps and sets: Complete 10 repetitions. Rest for thirty seconds to a minute and do a second set.

Progression 3

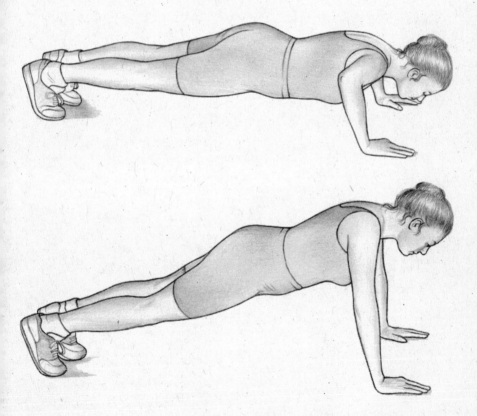

Focal points: Part of the difficulty of doing push-ups is holding your entire body in a straight line. This takes a lot of trunk strength. It may be helpful to have a friend tell you if your back is swayed or if you are holding your buttocks up. Don't forget to breathe while doing this challenging move!

EXERCISE 3: MID-BACK ◆

The middle of the back is an often overlooked and under-appreciated area. It is where I get many of my back problems stemming from my injury. The following series of progressions really targets the mid-back and helps with posture.

Progression 1: Butterfly Back
Starting position: Lie facedown on an exercise mat. Put your arms straight out at your sides, perpendicular to your body.

1-2-Pull: Contract your shoulder blades to lift your arms up and slightly back.

Hold your arms in the lifted position and draw four consecutive figure eights with your hands. (Each figure eight will take about three to four seconds.)

1-2-Down: Slowly relax your shoulders and arms back to the starting position.

Reps and sets: Complete 10 repetitions. Rest for thirty seconds to a minute and do a second set.

Progression 1

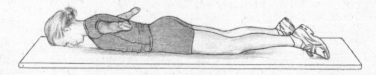

Focal points: When you are first starting, do the figure eights with your hands flat and palms down. But as you get comfortable with the exercise, try variations with the figure eights: Do them with your thumbs down, thumbs up, or pinkies up, or do them while holding a balled-up sock in each hand. The more you vary the movement, the more benefit you'll get because you'll be working slightly different muscle parts.

Progression 2: Seated Row
Starting position: Tie a knot in the middle of an exercise band and close a door on it so that you are on the side with the two ends hanging down and the knot is on the other side. Take care not to use a door that someone might open while you are doing the exercise. Sit in a chair facing the door, with good posture and feet flat on the floor, hip-width apart; the band should be at or slightly below shoulder level. Your arms will be out in front of your body at chest height, with palms facing down and elbows pointed out to the sides.

1-2-Pull: Slowly pull your hands toward your chest, keeping your elbows up and pointed out to the sides.

Pause for a moment.

1-2-3-Forward: Slowly relax your arms back to the starting position, keeping your elbows out to the sides.

Reps and sets: Complete 10 repetitions. Rest for thirty seconds to a minute and do a second set.

Progression 2

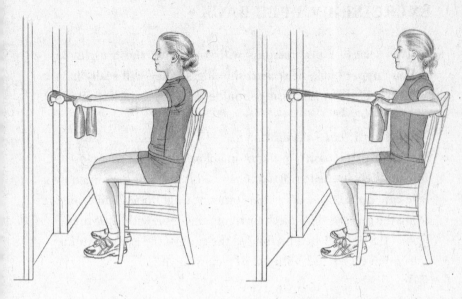

Focal points: Avoid locking your elbows between repetitions. Even though you are focusing on your arms and chest, don't forget to keep your trunk strong and supported by your abdominal muscles. Hold your shoulders down and back. Also, make sure that your hands and elbows are working on the same plane—at chest level.

Progressions: Increased Resistance
Do the same exercise with higher-resistance exercise bands to increase the difficulty. Work your way up through the three resistance levels: light, medium, and heavy. Be sure that you can maintain your form as you progress in resistance.

EXERCISE 4: UPPER BACK ◆

This series of progressions will strengthen the muscles in
your upper back, neck, and shoulders. They will really help
with posture by increasing shoulder and upper back strength.

Progression 1: Lateral Pull-down
Starting position: Tie a knot in an exercise band, and close the
knot securely in the top of a doorway with the ends hanging down.
Take care not to use a door that someone might open while you are
doing the exercise. Sit in a chair facing the door, with your toes
against the door. Reach up to hold the ends of the exercise tubing,
one end in each hand, with palms facing down.

1-2-Pull: Slowly pull your hands down and in toward your chest.
Keep your elbows pointed down, close to your body.

Pause for a moment.

1-2-3-Up: Slowly relax your arms back up to the starting position.

Reps and sets: Complete 10 repetitions. Rest for thirty seconds
to a minute and do a second set.

Focal points: As with the seated row, avoid locking your elbows
between repetitions. Keep your trunk stable and supported by your
abdominal muscles. Keep your shoulders broad, and think about
squeezing your shoulder blades together with each "pull."

Progressions: Increased Resistance
As this becomes easier for you, do the same exercise with higher-resistance exercise bands to increase the difficulty. Work your way up through the three resistance levels: light, medium, and heavy resistance. Be sure you can maintain your form as you progress in resistance.

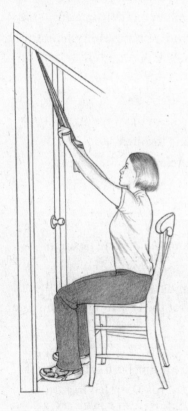

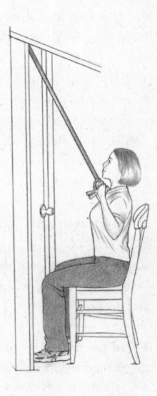

EXERCISE 5: LOWER BACK ◆

The lower back is the area that gives most people problems. Along with weak abdominal muscles, poorly trained back extensor muscles really contribute to back injuries and general lower back pain.

Progression 1: Superwoman
Starting position: Lie facedown on an exercise mat or carpet, or folded towel. Reach your right arm straight out in front of you on the floor with your palm down. Rest your left arm alongside your body, fingers pointing toward your toes, with palm up.

1-2-Up: Slowly, raise your right arm, chest, and left leg about 5 inches off the ground. Keep your face down (chin slightly tucked) so that your spine stays in a straight line through your neck. Your right leg and left hand should remain relaxed on the ground.

Pause for a moment.

1-2-3-Down: Relax your body back to the starting position.

Reps and sets: Complete 10 repetitions and then 10 repetitions on the other side; this is one set. Rest for thirty seconds to a minute and do a second set.

Focal points: Make sure that you are lifting both shoulders off the ground evenly, and keep your chest broad. Stretch from your fingertips through your toes to keep your body long and strong.

Progression 1

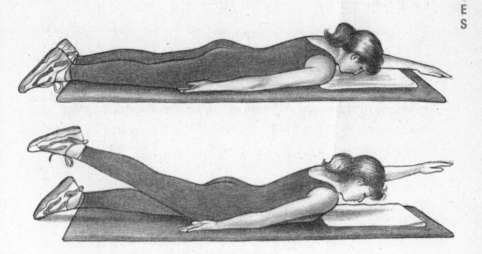

Progression 2: Bird Dog

Starting position: Kneel on all fours on an exercise mat, carpet, or folded towel, with the stability ball underneath your tummy. Your arms will be nearly straight (do not lock your elbows).

1-2-Up: Slowly, simultaneously raise your right arm straight out in front of you and your left leg straight out behind you. Use the ball to help balance yourself, but hold your trunk strong with abdominals contracted.

Pause for a moment.

1-2-3-Down: Slowly relax and lower your arm and leg back to the starting position.

Reps and sets: Complete 10 repetitions and then 10 repetitions on the other side; this is one set. Rest for thirty seconds to a minute and do a second set.

Focal points: This movement takes a lot of balance, which comes from strength. It may be difficult at first, but as you become stronger, your balance will improve and you will quickly find it becomes easier. If it is too hard to fully extend your arm/leg to start, just lift your arm and leg as much as you can.

Progression 2

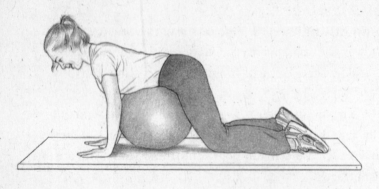

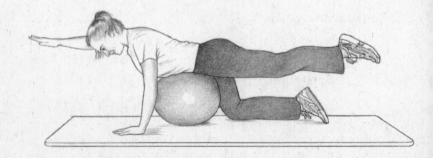

Progression 3: Back Extension

Starting position: Place an exercise mat with the short side against a wall. Kneel down on the mat with your feet flat against the wall (the tips of your toes touching the mat). Place the stability ball in front of you and lean your torso over it so that your back is nearly parallel to the floor. Cross your arms over your chest and use the wall to help keep your feet anchored.

1-2-Up: Slowly lift your upper body, keeping your pelvis pressed into the ball. Your body should be in a straight line from head to knees; take care not to overextend past this point.

Pause for a moment.

1-2-3-Down: In a controlled motion, lower your torso back down onto the ball.

Reps and sets: Complete 10 repetitions. Rest for thirty seconds to a minute and do a second set.

Focal points: Concentrate on using your back muscles to lift your torso, not your legs. And while it may be difficult, it is important to hold your head in a straight line with your spine. The lift movement doesn't seem very significant, but it isn't easy! When your torso is lifted, hold your back and tummy strong so that there is not a scoop in your back.

Progression 3

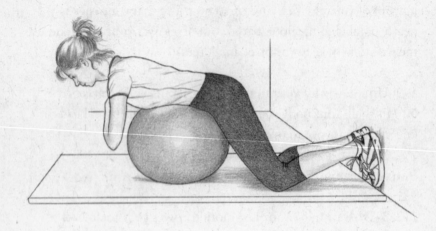

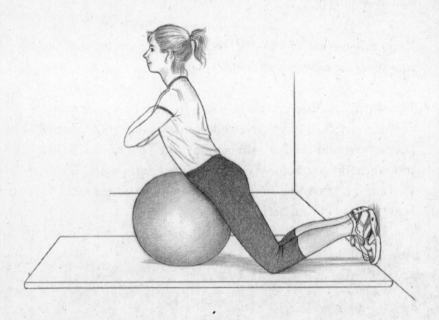

EXERCISE 6:
WALL SQUAT WITH STABILITY BALL ◆

Once you are comfortable with the first five exercises of the program and need a greater challenge, try adding this sixth exercise to your routine. It is a more complex move that targets many muscles in the trunk and hips. It also focuses on stability and posture. You can do it at work or at home while watching the evening news.

Starting position: Standing with a wall behind you, place a stability ball between your lower back and the wall. You will be leaning against the ball, with your feet greater than hip-width apart and slightly in front of your hips. Keep your arms straight out in front or crossed over your chest.

1-2-3-Down: While leaning against the ball, slowly bend at the knees as the ball rolls down the wall with your movement. Squat down only as far as is comfortable. The ball should now be at about your mid-back.

Pause for a moment.

1-2-Up: Keeping pressure against the ball, contract your buttocks and slowly "roll" yourself back up to the starting position.

Reps and sets: Complete 10 repetitions. Rest for thirty seconds to a minute and do a second set.

Focal points: The "squat" does not need to be a big movement to reap the benefit. In fact, if you squat too low, you may feel some pain in your knees (in which case you should stop). It may take a few tries to get the sense of placement for this exercise—where to place the ball on your lower back to start, and how far out to place your feet. In the squatting position, your knees should be directly over your toes. If your knees pass in front of your toes, then start with your feet slightly further out. Conversely, if you can still clearly see your toes when squatting, start with your feet slightly closer in.

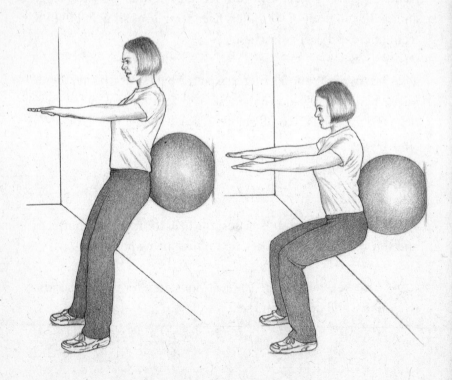

Strength Training: Fitness Center Alternatives

You may sometimes prefer doing your exercises at a fitness center. While the atmosphere proves discouraging for some, for others it is motivating. It all depends on your own tastes and proclivities.

If you do use a fitness center for your strength training, it will provide you the opportunity to do the moves on exercise mats, with the directions I have given in the previous pages, *or* to use weight machines. Doing a mix of exercising at home and at the gym, using both mats and machines, can help keep things interesting. Variation is a great way to continually stimulate your muscles and prevent boredom.

Speak to a fitness professional at your gym before using the machines for the first time. Ask her or him to show you the correct body positions, how to use the machines safely, and how to adjust the settings. It can be very educational, as well as confidence building, to schedule a training session with a personal trainer to help you get familiar with the equipment and show you proper form.

The bottom line, of course, is that you should do your workout wherever you feel inspired and wherever you know you will make it part of your routine. If you are in the mood to hit the gym, here are the alternatives for the strength-training portion of the program.

	EXERCISE	FITNESS CENTER ALTERNATIVE
1.	Abdominal Exercises	Abdominal Curl Machine
2.	Chest Muscle Exercises	Chest Press Machine
3.	Mid-back Exercises	Seated Row Machine
4.	Upper Back Exercises	Lateral Pull-down Machine (or Pull-up Bar)
5.	Lower Back Exercises	Back Extension (Machine or Bench)
6.	Wall Squat with Ball	Hack Squat or Smith Machine Squat

Flexibility Training

What is back flexibility? It means the muscles, tendons, and ligaments in your spine become more Gumby-like, if you will, more supple. That makes you able to twist and turn with much less risk of injury.

In order to make your back more flexible, you need to push it past its current range of motion. It takes time, but increased flexibility will eventually lead to greater freedom of movement, not to mention fewer backaches and pains and a reduced risk of injury.

Before Starting

Be certain you're warmed up before stretching by doing it directly after strength training or an aerobic activity. You can also do it at any time of day as long as you've warmed up your muscles first with some light activity. If you go right into stretches without first having gotten that "glow" into your body, you won't achieve maximum gains—and can potentially hurt yourself. (Athletes need to stretch *before* exercising as well as after to minimize the risk of injury.)

Stretches may be a little uncomfortable at first, but they should never prove painful. Apply common sense. If you find your muscles quivering or if the pain really persists, you've overstretched.

Do each stretch two times. The move should be slow and deliberate. It should be static, too. This means you should not bounce when you are fully stretched. Just hold the stretch at the point where you feel tight—but not hurting.

If you can stretch every single day, so much the better. That'll bring the greatest gains in flexibility.

HAMSTRING STRETCH ◆

Lie on your back on a mat or carpeted floor with knees bent. Lift your right leg up. With one end of an exercise band in each hand, reach your hands up and place the middle of the band over the middle of your foot. Keeping your knees slightly relaxed (not locked), adjust your hands on the band until there is some tension. Slowly pull your leg up toward your chest until you feel the stretch in the back of your right thigh. Stretch only as far as you can while maintaining a nearly straight leg; it should feel tight but comfortable. Hold for twenty seconds. Then do the stretch using your left leg. Complete the stretch two times on each leg. When you are ready, increase the hold time to thirty seconds or more.

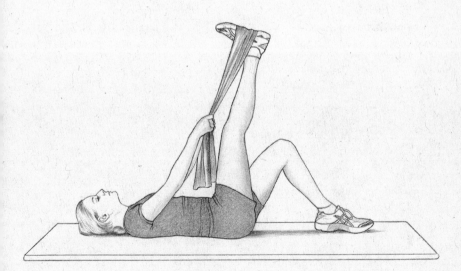

MULTI-BACK STRETCH ◆

This is a combination stretch. Curl up in a ball with your knees tucked under you and your arms stretched out in front of your head. Gently lean into the floor and hold for fifteen seconds. Now, get on your hands and knees with your back parallel to the floor. Your body will form a box. Round up your back like a cat and hold for fifteen seconds. Next, curve your back down to make a U and hold for an-

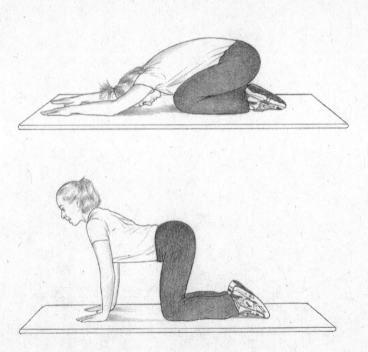

other fifteen seconds. Now, lie on your stomach with your legs stretched out behind you. Place your hands on the ground and push your chest up and hold for fifteen seconds. Each series of stretches takes about a minute to complete. Rest. Then repeat the entire combination of stretches.

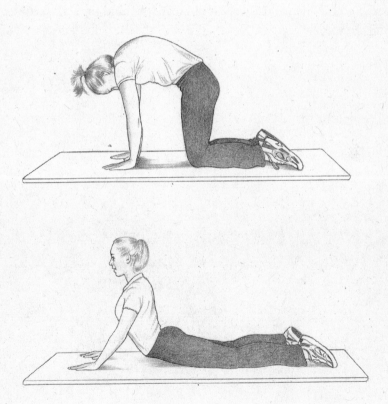

HIP EXTENSION STRETCH ◆

Get down on your right knee on a mat (left foot flat on the mat), with your hands on your hips. Move your left foot forward until it is well in front of your left knee. Now, slide your pelvis forward as far as you can. It is very important that you keep your hips square, and your left thigh should be parallel to the floor. Feel the stretch on the front of your right hip and thigh. Then do the stretch kneeling on your left leg.

Complete the stretch two times on each side, with twenty seconds per stretch. When you are ready, increase the hold time to thirty seconds or more.

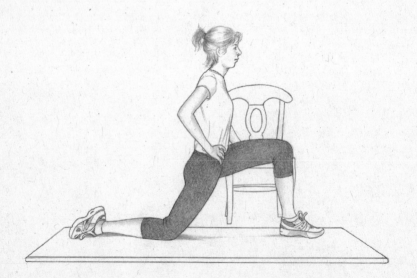

SIDE STRETCH ◆

Stand with your feet hip-width apart, with your right arm extended over your head (left arm hanging by your side). Now, bend at your side to reach your right arm over to the left as far as you can. Be sure to keep your body in a flat plane from side to side (avoid bending forward). Feel the stretch through the right side of your body. Then do the stretch on the other side.

Complete the stretch two times on each side, with twenty seconds per stretch. When you are ready, increase the hold time to thirty seconds or more.

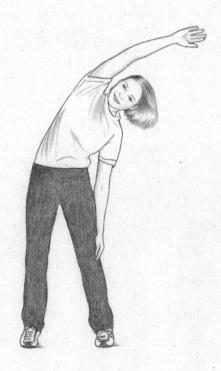

NECK STRETCH ◆

Sit in a chair with a tall, straight back. With your right arm relaxed at your side, reach up with your left hand to *gently* pull your head to the left side. You should feel the stretch through the right side of your neck. As you hold your head to the side, keep your shoulder down and back to deepen the stretch. Hold for twenty seconds. Now, by making a small adjustment, you will feel the stretch in a different place: use your left hand to pull your head slightly down to the front left side. You should feel the stretch on the back right side of your neck. Hold for twenty seconds. Then switch to stretch the other side of your neck.

Complete the stretch two times on each side, with twenty seconds per stretch. When you are ready, increase the hold time to thirty seconds or more.

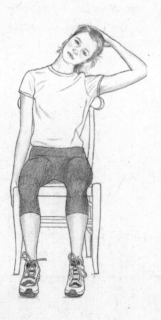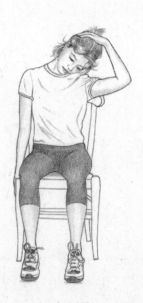

The Aerobic Factor

Aerobic exercise directly targets the heart, lungs, and the rest of the cardiovascular system. Those are the components of the body that are most challenged—and most rewarded—by aerobic activities such as brisk walking, jogging, swimming, and bicycling. Of course, aerobics also contributes to increasing endurance in whatever muscles are used to do the exercise—the leg muscles in walking, the arm muscles in rowing, both the arms and legs in swimming. So why is there an aerobic component to a program meant to strengthen the back?

One reason is that the back muscles are used in every kind of aerobic exercise, even if they're not the main muscles being used. So contributing to overall health in other parts of the body also means contributing to back health. Just as important, aerobic exercise helps to burn calories and is therefore crucial to long-term weight control, which in turn is crucial for keeping undue pressure off the back.

If you haven't been engaging in regular aerobic exercise for a long time, don't shoot for thirty minutes at a time at first. What's more important is consistency. Better to walk for ten minutes five days a week than to knock yourself out for two days by going for a half hour and then slacking off because you found it too difficult or too tiring. Soon enough—within weeks, in fact—you'll gradually be able to increase your efforts, say, by five minutes at a time, or at least five minutes a week.

Don't tell yourself not to bother because you can't accomplish much at your current fitness level. Everyone has to start somewhere. And if you start, I guarantee you'll keep getting better at it. In fact, within six weeks, your efforts will make you feel more energetic rather than tired out. The body adapts pretty quickly.

One way to begin is not to start with a formal aerobics program per se but to tuck more aerobic activity into your everyday routine to get you acclimated. For instance, try those tips that you always hear but that most people never do: park away from the mall or super-market entrance and walk the length of the parking lot; always use the stairs rather than take an escalator or elevator; walk to a store that's within reasonable walking distance rather than drive.

It might not sound like much, but you can easily burn 100 extra calories a day that way if you keep at it—enough to lose 10 pounds in a year's time if you don't add more calories.

After a couple of weeks of inserting little bursts of aerobics into your day, you'll find that starting a formal aerobics routine will be easier. Many people choose walking because there's no learning curve; everyone already knows how to do it. Walking is great (as long as you do it as if you are late for an appointment rather than window shopping), but if you'd prefer swimming, bicycling, Jazzercise, or working out with a dance exercise video in your own living room, then do that. Cross-country ski machines, elliptical trainers, stair climbers, and stair-stepping machines are fine, too. Choose what you really enjoy; you'll be more likely to stick with it. You can cross-train, too, if that helps you stay with it. Do some brisk walking on some days and a different aerobic exercise on others.

If you swim, ride a bike, or use a stationary rowing machine, cross-training becomes more important. None of those activities are weight-bearing, meaning you don't need your legs to carry the weight of your body while doing it. And you want to engage in at least some activities that require you to carry your weight, such as brisk walking or jogging, because those are the ones that help maintain the strength of your bones.

Goal: Thirty minutes or more, most days of the week.

Warm Up and Cool Down
Before you begin your aerobic activity, always warm up your body first by engaging in three to five minutes of low-intensity moves,

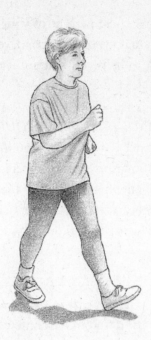

such as walking, dancing, or riding on a stationary bike. Most in-juries occur because the muscles and connective tissue are thrown into action too fast.

You should also cool down at the end of an aerobic exercise rather than stop abruptly. That eases pressure on your cardiovascular system by returning your heart rate and blood pressure *gradually* to their resting states. Five minutes of doing the exercise at a less intense pace makes a good cooldown. (The warm-up and cooldown can be part of your thirty-minute sessions. You don't have to tack them on.)

How Hard to Go At It

You should never do aerobic exercise as fast or as hard as you can, which would be as fast as your heart can possibly beat. Instead, aerobics should occur at 60 to 80 percent of your heart's fastest rate. That's rigorous enough to do your body good, yet safe.

There's an equation to help you figure out 60 to 80 percent of your maximum heart rate:

MAXIMUM HEART RATE = 220 MINUS YOUR AGE
Then figure 60 to 80 percent of the maximum. The equation isn't perfect, as there is variation from person to person. But it's a reasonable way of assessing whether you're going at the right intensity.

The chart below gives heart rates—beats per minute—for 60, 70, 80, and 90 percent intensity for ages 20 through 80 at five-year intervals.

	Heart rate in beats per minute at different percents of maximum			
AGE	60%	70%	80%	90%
20	120	140	160	180
25	117	137	156	176
30	114	133	152	171
35	111	130	148	167
40	108	126	144	162
45	105	123	140	158
50	102	119	136	153
55	99	116	132	149
60	96	112	128	144
65	93	109	124	140
70	90	105	120	135
75	87	102	116	131
80	84	98	112	126

EXERCISE INTENSITY SCALE
FOR AEROBIC TRAINING

EXERCISE INTENSITY LEVEL	DESCRIPTION OF EFFORT
1—Sedentary	No perceived effort: standing, sitting, or lying down.
2—Active This level contributes to overall health and burns more calories than being sedentary.	Easy, sustainable movement that causes a small increase in heart and breathing rate and doesn't raise a sweat (unless the weather is hot): strolling, gardening, slow dancing, golfing.
3—Aerobic training You should exercise at this level to condition your heart and lungs.	Somewhat hard movement that elevates the heart rate to 60 to 70 percent of maximum most of the time, ranging up to 80 percent. Breathing is more rapid, though it's possible to converse with only slightly altered speech; perspiration appears after about five to fifteen minutes, depending on air temperature.
4—Athletic training This is a more advanced level of aerobic conditioning that might become an appropriate goal after the 16-week program.	Hard effort that elevates the heart rate to 70 to 80 percent most of the time, ranging up to 90 percent of maximum. Breathing is more rapid but not labored—it's possible to converse, though faster breathing will cause evident interruptions; perspiration starts within five to ten minutes, depending on air temperature; fatigue will increase as the workout continues, and you will feel a need to stop by the end.
5—Overexertion Not recommended!	Excessive effort: heart pounds to the point of discomfort or nausea; breathing is too rapid to permit speech.

TARGET HEART RATE = 60 to 80 percent
of MAXIMUM HEART RATE

Of course, once you determine your range for your target heart rate, you need to be able to figure out whether you're in that range while you're actually exercising. You can do that by taking your pulse and seeing whether you're heart is pumping at 60 to 80 percent of its maximum capacity, but an easier method is to use an intensity scale.

With the intensity scale here, you should shoot for level 3, sometimes going up to level 4. That means that *for most of the exercise, you should be able to more or less keep up a conversation yet at some points be able to complete only a sentence here and there.* If you can't get out more than a word or two at a time, you're pushing yourself too hard—above 90 percent of your maximum heart rate—and you won't be able to sustain the effort. For some it may even be dangerous.

STAYING ON TOP OF IT

Research has shown repeatedly that keeping an exercise log makes people much more likely to stick to their plan. It forces you to reckon with yourself—as well as shows you your accomplishments in black and white, which helps keep you going.

I have written an entire book, *The Strong Women's Journal,* that allows women to keep careful exercise (and eating) records, but you can also use the exercise log here. Just make a bunch of photocopies and keep them all in one place.

STRENGTH TRAINING Goal: 3 times per week			
EXERCISE 2 SETS/10 REPS	DAY: "√"	DAY: "√"	DAY: "√"
Abdominals			
Chest			
Mid-back			
Upper Back			
Lower Back			
Wall-squats			
FLEXIBILITY Goal: daily			
STRETCHES	"√"	"√"	"√"
Hamstring Stretch			
Multi-back			
Hip Extension			
Side Stretch			
Neck Stretch			

PLANNED AEROBIC ACTIVITY Goal: 6 times per week		
DAY	ACTIVITY	TIME

Comments:

COMBINING THE STRONG BACK PROGRAM WITH OTHER EXERCISES

This is a very concentrated back exercise program. I encourage you to do these moves for several months to really strengthen your back and improve flexibility. But after a while, you'll want to start adding other strength-training exercises into your program, both to keep boredom from setting in and to get your whole body strong. To do so, check out one of my other books; join a fitness center, where you'll be able to work out on resistance machines; hire a personal trainer for a few sessions to freshen up your routine. You can also learn several exercise routines by visiting www.strongwomen.com or getting some help at a health club. Even if you don't belong to a gym, many of them let you buy a day pass, and you can get strength-training tips from certified trainers on staff.

Josephine, the woman who attested to the benefits of exercise earlier in the chapter, says that once you get used to it, it's not a big deal at all. "I don't even do that much," she confesses, "about thirty minutes every other day. But the pain is definitely less. I have less tingling, too. I've really reduced the pain and increased my quality of life."

CHAPTER 5

Stress Reduction and Related Tactics *That Work*

◈

My back pain came in my third year of law school. I was 26 at the time and dealing with the stress of trying to finish summa cum laude and prepare for the bar exam. I was also unhappy because I was graduating and single and thought I would meet someone but hadn't. The pain got so bad that I got Reasonable Accommodation from the Americans with Disabilities Act to take the bar exam lying down in a private room because I couldn't sit in a chair.

It wasn't until after the bar, around the time I gave up on marriage and bought my own apartment and my own china and decided to concentrate on being a career woman, that my back pain went away. (So did my inability to find a mate. Once I "let go" and the stress receded, I met my future husband.)

—AMANDA

I t's true. Carrying the weight of the world on your shoulders, having a particularly difficult cross to bear, dealing with a yoke around your neck—whatever metaphor you want to use, emotional stress can go hand in hand with back pain.

The story of Amanda's emotional state bringing on her back pain is not unusual. For many people, emotional stress often exacerbates pain, makes it more persistent or harder to ignore, but it can also actually get it going. Stress's effects on the back run the gamut. The research on this topic is fascinating, showing that how we feel emotionally can have as much or more to do with physical pain as structural glitches in our bodies.

In a study conducted at Stanford University, researchers found that psychological distress may be a better predictor of lower back pain down the line than magnetic resonance imaging (MRI), which can identify cracks or tears in cartilage along with other structural problems. Following dozens of people for four years, the Stanford scientists discovered that the association between MRI findings and future back pain was not statistically significant. But what emerged clearly was that the subjects suffering psychological distress were three times more likely to develop back pain—and take medications for it and lose work days—than people with better coping skills. That is, psychosocial factors trumped the actual state of the back when it came to making a link to future lumbar spine pain.

In another research project conducted in Sweden, when investigators reviewed thirty-seven studies on possible predictors of back and neck pain, they identified a clear link with psychological variables. Those variables—stress, distress, and anxiety—were all found to be significant factors in back pain, related not only to the onset of pain but also to whether it was chronic rather than lasting just a short while.

In yet another study that took place in New Zealand, nursing students followed during their three years of training and for one year afterward were more likely to experience new episodes of lower back pain if they had preexisting psychological stress.

HOW STRESS CAN IMPACT THE BACK

What is it about emotional stress that can contribute to an actual physical reaction in the back?

One explanation is that as pain persists, a person becomes more anxious about performing daily activities, let alone exercise, for fear of worsening the discomfort. That, in turn, leads to physical deconditioning that makes the back more vulnerable to injury, which in turn leads to more pain—and more stress—thus creating a vicious cycle. Fear of using one's back can even lead to social isolation in extreme cases, thereby increasing the odds for emotional stress in the form of depression.

Stress also heightens pain's emotional component (yes, pain does have an emotional component). It diminishes overall coping ability and erodes one's sense of control over her life. Consequently, stress can make a person less likely to feel equipped to "take the reins" to do something to remedy back pain.

Another possibility is that emotional tension can cause changes in the body's nervous system, leading to muscle tension and eventual spasms. It certainly stands to reason that tension resulting from the stress of not being able to meet payroll, a job loss, divorce, or other negative life change can lead to tension in the spine. After all, we know that even everyday stress can make your muscles tighten. The longer lasting the tension and resultant muscle tightening, the greater the chances for ensuing pain.

Sometimes the pain of a physical insult to the back, perhaps via lifting something heavy the wrong way or a car accident, can continue even after the back has healed physically because, in the wake of an injury, negative emotions can be released that then linger.

GETTING THE STRESS OFF YOUR BACK

Whatever the reason for the mind/body connection that links stress to back pain, there are a number of avenues of relief. A couple of these avenues are completely nonphysical. They specifically help heal the back by way of the mind. Others involve types of exercise, or at least movements, that I have not yet discussed. They belong in this chapter rather than the previous one because research has linked them both to stress reduction *and* a stronger spine.

Nonphysical Approaches

Following are three lifestyle approaches that reach the back through the brain.

Meditation

People are often turned off by the idea of meditation. They think it means sitting cross-legged on the floor in a loincloth. It doesn't.

One psychologist has correctly described meditation as a "purely mechanical process" during which a person simply sits for twenty minutes a day with eyes closed. During that time, the meditator repeats a soothing sound that allows the body to settle down and release stress. (The soothing sound is one's mantra.) The result is a balance between the mind and the body.

That emotional health and physical health are inextricably interwoven is illustrated very well through the effects of meditation. It reduces heart rate and blood pressure and improves mood, all of which can indirectly lessen a back's burden. Far too many of us are not as meditative as we should be.

There are actually several types of meditation, all of which Western medicine refers to as types of *relaxation response.* Researchers believe part of what ties them together is their ability to inhibit the action of hormones that are involved in stress responses to pain.

Major cities in the United States have local meditation centers, often listed under Transcendental Meditation, where you can learn this relaxation technique. There are also a number of books on various types of meditation. One I highly recommend is Dr. Herbert Benson's *The Relaxation Response* (see Resources). A mind-body specialist with Harvard Medical School, Dr. Benson has pulled together aspects of different types of meditation that appear to significantly lower blood pressure—and other body markers associated with stress.

Psychotherapy

A psychiatrist, psychologist, social worker, or other mental health professional can be instrumental in helping you manage back pain. Consider that some people with long-lasting back problems develop an imbalance of neurotransmitters in the brain; pain can do that. And that, in turn, influences how pain signals are processed and interpreted. Working with a psychological counselor might help to retrain the brain by working through stresses that both contribute to and result from back pain.

For instance, sometimes a mental health worker can help because chronic pain leads to depression, which has to be treated along with the back pain itself. Treating the depression might not automatically lift the pain, but it can sometimes get someone to the point that she doesn't feel hopeless about working to get the back some relief.

Connecting with Others

Much of the reason my Tufts colleagues and I travel around the country all the time is to help others become what I call *agents of change*. That is, we work with people in various communities to become involved in leading exercise classes, fitness programs, and the like. And while it gets people more in shape, it also provides benefits that go well beyond that. When people are part of a larger community, when they come outside of themselves to take part in a group activity, they often are able to reorder their priorities in such a way that whatever was very troubling to them before is no longer as front and center.

I'm not suggesting that someone who suffers from back pain can make it fully dissipate by dint of getting out and seeing other people. But I have seen over and over that those who make a point of becoming involved in their communities are able to push problems that have been at the fore a little to the side, and that diminishes their impact. Becoming involved includes everything from joining a fitness group to working at a soup kitchen to volunteering at a library or after-school tutoring program. Your town newspaper or town hall probably has a listing of organizations that need people like you to share your strength one way or another.

Mind-Body Moves

The following exercises target the back via the brain and also directly. These mind-body moves can have powerful effects.

Tai Chi

A graceful martial arts form, tai chi is based, in large part, on an ancient Chinese martial art called tai chi quan, which requires tranquility and calmness while emphasizing slow, soft movements. Research in countries around the world has demonstrated that tai chi can reduce stress and improve back health.

Tai chi also helps the back at the site of the back itself. Many tai chi movements, which strengthen the core of the body, use the spine as a pivot. And that causes the spine and the muscles surrounding it to gently flex through tai chi poses with names like *White Crane Spreads Its Wings* and *Step Up to Seven Stars*. Through the repetition of such poses, the muscles around the spine, which include the abdominals and the back extensor muscles, become stronger. That then helps to improve posture and also reduce back pain; the better the strength and posture, the less slouching and rounding of the shoulders and the better the spinal alignment, which lessens stress on various spinal components.

Finally, tai chi helps lessen existing back pain by increasing flexibility.

The idea behind tai chi is to improve mind-body awareness with controlled yet fluid movements that focus on balance, breathing, and the body's place in its immediate environment as it moves through various positions and holds a variety of poses. Breathing is slow and deep as the trunk and limbs go through what are typically circular motions, intermingled with static poses. The aim is always on focusing your energy to get the most out of your strength and mental concentration—an inner stillness but with clarity. The deep breathing facilitates the process by encouraging oxygenated blood to flow to the muscles and brain.

One of the best things about tai chi is that it can be practiced by people who are otherwise sedentary. It also complements the main exercise program in this book really well.

A good tai chi class starts off at a level that is comfortable, then progresses to more difficult moves. It never jars the spine or any other part of the body.

Tai chi classes are offered in most geographic areas. Classes tend to be led by instructors at local community centers and Ys, and they're generally not expensive. Just be sure to check with your physician before you start.

Yoga

To practice yoga does not mean you have to be among the superflexible, double-jointed minority, turning yourself into a pretzel with circus-like agility. Indeed, millions of Americans of all levels of physical fitness practice yoga. Why?

It helps to reduce stress and enhance mood, which in turn makes back pain less *magnified* in one's life. Reduce the perception of pain, or the central importance of pain, and you in effect reduce the pain itself.

But practicing yoga isn't just about getting your head in a better place to take the focus off back pain. Similar to tai chi, it acts on the back itself, too. By increasing flexibility, range of motion, and muscle strength, and also by improving posture, balance, and coordination, practicing yoga can potentially go a long way to alleviate back problems, particularly problems of the lower back. Yoga can even help heal injured back muscles—and prevent reinjury.

The most popular kind of yoga in the United States is called *hatha* yoga, which involves a series of static postures, or *asanas,* that includes twisted positions and forward and backward bends. You hold each posture anywhere from ten to sixty seconds, flexing some muscles while relaxing others to allow both better conditioning and gradual destressing. Concentrated breathing exercises, called *pranayamas,* are also involved during the moves, helping the body and the mind get in sync by working to get both more supple. (None of this should be uncomfortable, but it does require concentration.)

Note that you don't have to be in great physical shape to derive benefits from yoga. In fact, there's a type of *hatha* yoga called *Iyengar* yoga that works well for people with physical limitations because it uses props like blocks, belts, and other supports to help achieve postures comfortably with a reduced risk for injury. One yoga expert I know teaches it to people ranging from age 50 to 90-plus who have a variety of chronic disabilities.

Fortunately, good yoga instructors are becoming easier to find these days, both at local Ys and fitness centers; however, deciding on one takes a gut feeling more than anything else because there is no national standardized credentialing program. I suggest you at least look for an instructor with several years' experience who understands your aims and limitations, preferably someone with a good fitness background, such as a degree in an exercise or fitness field or certification from a national, standardized organization, like the American Council on Exercise (ACE), the American College of Sports Medicine (ACSM), or the Aerobic and Fitness Association of America (AFAA). If the instructor pushes you to the point that it hurts, that's not good. (A few of the most common yoga postures, such as Cobra and Plough, can actually cause further injury in some people if performed too aggressively, so you want to be sure to discuss your condition with the instructor before class, and you want to be sure she or he is willing and able to modify the movements for you.) By the same token, if you don't feel any stretch or challenge in your muscles whatsoever, you're not being pushed to a point that you will derive much benefit.

Pilates

Like yoga and tai chi, Pilates (pih-LAH-teez) is all about a mind-body connection. It was developed in the early 1900s by a German man named Joseph Pilates, who was keenly aware that the brain influences the body's physiology. He learned from experience—as a weak child in poor health who so wanted to be fit and strong that he eventually managed to train himself to ski, box, do gymnastics, even become a circus performer.

Essentially, Pilates uses precise, controlled movements in the trunk to increase flexibility and strength in the abdomen, lower back, and pelvis—the body's core. Each movement is supposed to be performed with concentration and positive thought and with a deepening sensitivity to each and every part of the body. The result is not only better conditioning and a better frame of mind (breathing is used to promote focusing and "centering"), but better posture, too, which takes undue pressure off various parts of the spine.

Pilates classes can be individual, with special Pilates equipment that uses springs to provide resistance for the movements, or group "mat classes" in which the moves are performed on padded floor mats. (These are much less expensive than the one-on-one classes with the specially designed equipment.)

If you do sign up for Pilates sessions or a group class and already have a serious back problem, speak to your physician first. Some of the moves may not be recommended for people with certain types of pain. Generally speaking, back patients should avoid moves that force the spine into extremes of extension, flexion, or twisting. Of course, if an exercise causes pain, stop. And don't be surprised if it takes a while for you to fully realize the benefits of a Pilates program; it takes time to reprogram old muscle "memory" and tap the strength of previously underutilized trunk muscles.

Twenty years ago, hardly anyone had even heard of Pilates. Today, it's practiced by many millions of people. It is an exercise that I myself would like to do more of.

Other Methods to Consider

While yoga, tai chi, and Pilates involve your own movement, there are also some techniques in which *others* make the movements on your back. They can go a long way toward healing the spine, and they decrease stress, too.

Massage

In a study conducted at the University of Miami, it was found that massage therapy lessened lower back pain, not only by acting directly on the back but also by working on the brain. Specifically, it reduced depression and anxiety and improved sleep, all of which may have contributed to the beneficial effect.

Researchers at Seattle's Group Health Cooperative made a similar finding when they followed some 260 people, most of whom had been having low back pain continuously for a year or more. Those who received ten weeks of massage therapy suffered less disability than others. They did not have as much difficulty going up stairs, turning over in bed, or putting on their clothes. They also filled less pain medication prescriptions than back sufferers who didn't receive massage therapy, and they tallied up a lower price tag for outpatient HMO back services.

Massage is thought to work directly on the back by improving blood circulation and relaxing muscles, leading to an improved range of motion. The soft tissue manipulation can also reduce pain and improve one's ability to move around. And it can loosen up tightened muscles or relieve muscle spasms. In addition, some massage therapists encourage their clients to stretch and exercise, which could ameliorate back pain in themselves.

As for the lessening of depression and other contributors to emotional stress, it is thought that massage may lead to increased levels of endorphins—"feel-good" chemicals in the brain. Of course, spending an hour or so in a quiet environment could also help, as might being touched in a therapeutic context. Both can ratchet down stress levels, which in turn can work to relax overly tight muscles.

The type of massage said to be helpful for alleviating muscle aches that may be involved in back pain is not Swedish massage, which is gentle and lulling. It's a more aggressive massage, either in the form of deep-tissue massage, myofascial release, neuromuscular facilitation, or Rolfing. The first three types are all meant to stretch muscles and connective tissue (known as fascia) with the application of steady, even, and, at times, very firm pressure. Neuromuscular massage, in particular, applies strong pressure to painful knots or spasms in the muscles. Rolfing "reeducates" the body about posture by realigning the back with other areas through working the connective tissue that surrounds the muscles. (The most highly trained practitioners are taught at the Rolf Institute of Structural Integration, in Boulder, Colorado. See Resources.)

All of these types of massage can feel somewhat painful and can even cause some residual soreness that lasts up to a day to a day and a half. They should never be overly painful, however. People tend to describe their effects as "good pain."

Note that massage is best thought of as *adjunctive* therapy for back pain. It generally doesn't completely eliminate pain on its own. Also, it is not the best treatment for *inflamed* muscles or pinched nerves. People considering massage therapy should see a physician to make sure any physical cause for their back pain does not make massage ill-advised.

To increase the odds that you will be choosing a qualified massage therapist, inquire how many years the person has been in practice and what her or his particular specialties are. Check for the initials

NCTMB after her or his name, too. That signifies that the massage therapist has passed a thorough examination to become certified by the National Certification Board for Therapeutic Massage and Body-work. You should also ask whether she or he has graduated from a training program accredited or approved by the Commission on Massage Therapy Accreditation. Twenty-nine states regulate massage therapists as well, so you can often check to see that yours is licensed. (Some states license town by town.) Note, however, that the standards set in many states are soft, and the organizations involved may promote some fringe ideas about massage's benefits. Consider that the Commission on Massage Therapy Accreditation standards do not require that teachings be scientifically valid.

Finally, check to see whether your health insurer will pay for the sessions. In some cases, massage therapy may be covered.

Feldenkrais Method

More than half a century ago, a Russian-born physicist named Moshe Feldenkrais, who also happened to be a black belt in judo as well as a soccer player, had a knee injury that was so bad it was expected to interfere with his ability to walk. To recover, he applied his scientific mind to the job of thinking through the mechanics of the body and brain in a way he could make use of. The result, arrived at in the 1940s, was what is now known as the Feldenkrais method.

Essentially, what Feldenkrais theorized was that as children our movements are right for our bodies but that as we age we "learn" movements that limit our coordination, range of motion, and body awareness, in turn causing undue stress on various parts of our skeletons. Simply put, we learn to move in a way that involves a great deal of unnecessary muscle tension, and that leads to a lot of unnecessary pain.

The way around it is body, or movement "education," literally teaching people how to move more efficiently, with all the body parts working in sync. A Feldenkrais instructor takes a person's neuro-muscular system, largely through touch, through precise movements that are meant to change habitual patterns. The touch is meant as guidance rather than a form of therapy. The teacher gently lifts and supports the back, chest, and other body parts while talking the student through slow movements that are not taxing to the body. The end result is not only an education about how to move in a way that will support the back better but also better body awareness, less stress on the joints, an increased range of motion, and a sense of re-laxation and well-being.

Unfortunately, there are few scientific studies confirming or denying the usefulness of the Feldenkrais Method, so claims for bet-ter health are mostly anecdotal (although a few research efforts sug-gest relief from back pain). But the anecdotal evidence is strong enough to warrant consideration.

Some Feldenkrais instructors work specifically with people who have orthopedic or neurologic conditions that contribute to pain or limit movement—arthritis or whiplash, for instance. Others work to relieve pain in athletes or performers such as dancers and musicians.

Some teachers guide a group of students in a classroom setting; others go one–on–one in a process called functional integration, with the student lying fully clothed on a table while the instructor uses gentle touch combined with verbal suggestions to insure that no joint is being stressed more than it needs to be.

You don't have to be a health care professional to be a Feldenkrais instructor, although many physical therapists and massage thera-pists are Guild-certified practitioners. If you want to learn the Felden-krais method, look for a practitioner who has been certified by the Feldenkrais Guild of North America (see Resources). Note that unless Feldenkrais sessions are conducted by a health care professional licensed in a profession such as physical therapy, they most likely will not be covered by insurance.

Alexander Technique
Just as the Feldenkrais Method works to integrate the mind and the body to reduce stress in movement as well as promote a sense of well-being, so does the Alexander Technique. It was invented by Frederick Alexander, an Australian actor born in the 1860s who went through bouts of hoarseness while performing. Neither medications nor rest helped him, but using mirrors, he was able to see that the way he lowered his head and tensed his neck muscles while speaking his lines served to restrict his vocal cords. He corrected his posture, his voice came back to normal, and the Alexander Technique was born.

The idea behind it is that the correct alignment of the head, neck, and spine are crucial to good health. As such, the aim of the technique, which like the Feldenkrais Method uses verbal instruction and gentle touch, is to do away with counterproductive postural habits like slouching and tensing. Muscle tension is relieved, too, and movement is made easier. Even emotional stress can diminish to some degree; if the body is less tense, so is the mind.

Gold standard clinical proof for the Alexander Technique is lacking, but research *has* suggested relief for chronic back pain sufferers, and scoliosis patients treated with it strengthened the muscles in their spine as well as improved their physical appearance. Today, many performing arts schools incorporate the Alexander Technique for their students. (My husband, a violinist, has practiced it himself—and the music school he teaches at also offers courses in the Feldenkrais Method.)

If you want to try it, find an instructor who is certified by the North American Society of Teachers of the Alexander Technique.

(Alexander Technique International in Cambridge, Massachusetts, can refer you to one. See Resources.) To earn certification, instructors must complete at least three years of training.

DON'T IGNORE THE MIND-BODY CONNECTION

The approaches I list here represent many, but not all, of the ways that people can work to minimize back pain by getting at both emotional stress and stress on the spine. There are also techniques such as guided imagery, self-hypnosis, and progressive muscle relaxation (all of which involve relaxation responses). A trusted mental health counselor should be able to tell you more about them.

Whichever mode(s) you choose, do choose something if you want to prevent or alleviate back pain and are experiencing ongoing stress. A good exercise program is crucial, to be sure. But minimizing your stress really will go a long way to ease your back's burden.

CHAPTER 6

Are You Ergonomically Correct? Making Your Environment More Back Friendly

◈

Twenty years ago, when I first came to Tufts, I moved into a brand-new research facility that, at the time, was state-of-the-art. It was a clean, streamlined building, and many offices, including mine, had panoramic views over Boston. But my work space wasn't right for my body. At my height, five feet four inches (if I exaggerate a bit!), most desks and chairs were just too high for me. Furthermore, the relative heights and distances of my chair, desk, and computer to one another weren't adjustable to my small frame. Even after propping a box under my feet, my neck was often strained and my back uncomfortable.

Then, three years ago, I moved over to a just-completed research building one block away from the other one. My window now faces the side of a brick building directly across the street. But what I have lost in view I have gained in comfort. So has everyone else who has moved into this new building. Every desk and chair has been ergonomically designed so that they can be adjusted to accommodate each person's body size. No more boxes under my feet. No more neck strain. No more back pain as I work.

My administrative assistant loves that she can adjust her desk height so that she can work *standing* if she wants, in order not to put too much stress on any one muscle group in her spine or neck. Her thinking is right. Changing positions periodically is just what people who specialize in ergonomics recommend in order for various parts of the body to get a break here and there. In other words, our new offices are ergonomically correct.

What *is* ergonomics, anyway? People bandy the term about, but few can define it.

Ergonomics is the science that concerns itself with the interface between humans and other elements of a "system," such as an office. The better that interface, the more efficiently and productively the human and the system will work together. The term "ergonomics" is derived from the Greek *ergon* (for work) and *nomos* (laws), which means, loosely translated, the laws of science that govern work.

It might seem that ergonomics wouldn't be terribly important to me. After all, I'm a very active person who exercises almost every single day and is often on the road *promoting* exercise, meaning that I spend a fair amount of time away from my desk. But most people, no matter how active they are, spend much of their workday sedentary. The reality is that for many hours each weekday I am either sitting at my desk working on the computer or talking on the phone—or sitting in a conference room, or on an airplane. That's true for most people. Unless you work in retail or manufacturing (and those people tend to spend a lot of time in one position, too, which I'll get to later), about a third of every twenty-four hours tends to get spent sitting, often in one place. That's a lot of pressure on the back, particularly the vulnerable lower back, which is why it's so important that your work space be ergonomically correct. It's important not just for the comfort of your back and neck but of your whole body.

Roughly another third of each day is spent in bed, and another third in places where your spine is also at work, even if the rest of you is not—the car, the kitchen, the family room. That's why this chapter is broken up into three main sections: one devoted to the ergonomics of your work space, another to your bed, and a third to the ergonomics involved in your activities outside of work and sleep.

If your ergonomics are right, you won't be unduly tilting your pelvis and shifting your spine, putting added pressure on muscles and joints there. You won't be hunched over as you type or prepare meals in your kitchen. You won't be straining your shoulders as you carry your head (a fairly heavy part of your body). Rather, you'll be in "neutral," meaning that your spine will be in its natural curvature as much as possible—a position that allows you to complete your tasks without undue stress on any one particular part of the body.

YOUR WORK ENVIRONMENT

You might say that there are two kinds of people: those whose work predominately involves sitting and those whose work entails a lot of standing. As such, their ergonomic needs are different. Here is a rundown:

If You Sit Most of the Day

For those who spend most of the workday behind a desk, the object is to allow your body into a position that doesn't strain it. That is, your work space should accommodate you. No part of your body should have to stretch, tilt, bend, or constrict unnecessarily to accommodate your desk, chair, or computer screen or keyboard. Otherwise, you're setting yourself up for strain not just on the muscles in your back and neck but also the rest of the skeleton. And such strain, over many hours each day and then through the months and years, leads to pain.

Consider the following elements of sitting properly, and refer to the illustration. Good sitting will distribute weight evenly throughout the spinal column; open the diaphragm to allow for the fullest breathing; and even aid digestion by leaving the lower part of the abdomen unconstricted.

- While typing or writing, your hands, wrists, and forearms (lower arms) should all be in a straight line and pretty much parallel to the floor.
- Your head should be directly above your neck, or bent forward slightly (but no more than 20 degrees). It should essentially be in line with your torso. If it is jutting out or leaning back, something about your work station—or your work posture—is off. (Because the head is relatively heavy, you don't want it pulling unduly on any of your back muscles.)
- Your shoulders should be *relaxed*. That doesn't mean slumping, but you should not have to feel stiff or tight in your shoulders as you go about your duties.
- Your elbows should be close to your body. There shouldn't be a sense of flapping as you work.
- Your feet should be *fully* on the floor—or on a flat footrest.
- Sit back in your chair as you work, not on its edge. Your chair should support your spine all along its length, particularly in the small of your back—the lumbar region. That's true

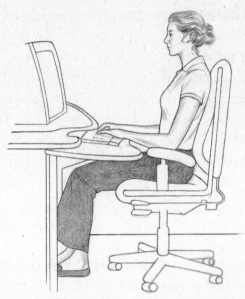

whether you're sitting up straight or leaning back a little (as you're talking on the phone, for instance).

- Your knees should be at about the same height as your hips, and your feet should come forward a little.

Now, how best to align your desk and chair so that your equipment, rather than you, bears the brunt of the workload for you to remain in the proper position?

1. Adjust your seat's height so that your hip is just a little bit higher than your knee. (If your feet don't reach the floor this way, you must put them flat on a footrest.)
2. Make sure that when your forearms are parallel to the floor, your desk height is level with your elbows. (If the desk if too low, raise it by putting something under its legs. If it's too high, raise your chair height and use a footrest, if necessary.)

3. Keep your computer monitor directly in front of you and at least 20 inches away from you (but generally not more than 40 inches). The top line of the screen should be at or below eye level. This will prevent eye strain in addition to preventing back pain. If your screen is too far away, you will have to lean forward to see and lose the support of your chair's backrest. And if the screen is too close, you may have to tilt your head back and place undue tension on your neck, shoulders, and spine.

Note: It may not always be possible to keep your monitor directly in front of you, particularly if you are working off printed material. If that's the case, it's okay to keep the monitor up to 35 degrees to one side and put the printed matter directly in front of you. Always keep the printed materials and the monitor as close to each other as possible.

Making Your Office Equipment Work for You

Obviously, not every desk, chair, and computer monitor and keyboard are going to be automatically aligned so that your body is in the best position to keep strain off your back. That's why it's critical that the equipment in your work space be adjustable. Answer the following questions to assess your office space's adjustability. The more you can answer with a "yes," the better your work space can be altered to accommodate the needs of your particular body. (And the more likely you will be to do the altering. Research on office ergonomics has shown that the quicker and easier it is to adjust your office components, the greater the chance that you'll save your body by putting the equipment to work.)

Chair

1. Is the chair height adjustable so that the entire length of your feet can rest comfortably on the floor?
2. Can the height of the chair back be adjusted independently from the seat?
3. Can the chair back recline in case you want to lean back a little while talking on the phone or taking a break?
4. Can the seat itself be tilted forward or backward?
5. Are the controls for adjusting chair height and seat tilt and height easy to use and within easy reach so that you'll change positions when you need to, rather than not make a necessary adjustment because it's just too hard?
6. Does your chair swivel 360 degrees so that you can face anywhere you want in it without straining?

Desk

1. Is it possible to adjust your desk height? Some desks and worktables are electronically adjustable, which allows people to stand for part of the day as they work, if they prefer. And many do prefer that. In a Cornell University study, in fact, most people with access to adjustable-height computer workstations chose to work while standing for about 20 percent of the day. (They also reported less upper-body discomfort, less afternoon discomfort, and more productivity than people who did not have access to adjustable-height workstations.)
2. Does your desk have enough surface area so that your papers—and you—are not cramped over one too small spot as you are trying to work?

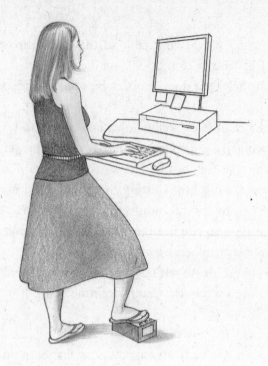

Computer Monitor

1. Can you tilt your monitor up or down?
2. Is your monitor able to swivel to the left and right? (Glare on the screen from sunlight at certain times of the day could have you straining your back if you're not able to adjust the position a little.)
3. Are you able to change the height of your screen?
4. Can you move the screen closer or further away so that it's 20 to 40 inches away from you? (In some cases, you may have to move the desk forward from the wall a little to make room for the back of the monitor. Flat-screen monitors can start out farther back than traditional ones.)
5. Can you easily change the resolution on your screen so that

you're not squinting, which is often done while the back is hunched over?

Keyboard

1. Is there room on the keyboard to support and rest your wrists? If the keyboard comes right to the edge of the desk, you will be squishing yourself—and your back and shoulder muscles. You should be able to rest your hands comfortably so that your wrists are in a neutral position as you type—a straight line from elbow to fingertips.

2. Is the keyboard tray height-adjustable? Does it have what is known as a negative slope, meaning it can tilt away from you? Those keyboard trays whose heights can adjust down toward your lap and allow you to tilt them away from your body work best. They allow the body and hands to maintain the most neutral working position, without any undue pressure on the spine.

3. If your keyboard has a wrist rest, is it broad and flat and relatively firm? Soft, gel-filled wrist rests will contour to your wrist and therefore allow for wrist twisting—not good. You may not need any wrist rest at all. Despite wrist rests' popularity these days, there is no research to indicate a benefit. Try typing with and without one, and choose whichever way feels better to you.

Note that most ergonomic keyboards sold today are split, with the alphabet and numeric keys on an angle. While that prevents overworking the wrists to some degree, there is no clear research that shows it offers any postural benefits. For most people, a regular keyboard works fine as long as it's placed in a position that allows your wrists to remain level with your forearm.

Phone Talk

Many people, including me, spend a good deal of each day on the phone. Often, rather than hold the phone in their hands, which they need to do to type or write or turn pages as they speak, they hold it in place at the neck by squeezing their head against a shoulder. All that crimping of the neck and shoulder muscles is a perfect setup for pain. That's why it's really important to have your hands free for other tasks during a phone conversation.

One solution is using a speakerphone. But many people on the other end don't like the hollowness they often hear on the line during speakerphone conversations. They also don't like the feeling that anybody walking by or in the room can hear whatever they say. To get around those issues, I've invested in a hands-free headset. It feels a little funny to put it on your head at first, but during the first long phone conversation in which you have to type or turn pages, you'll never look back. If your employer doesn't spring for hands-free headsets, you can buy one for less than $100 in any small-appliance store. You may not want to shell out the money, but your spine, neck, and shoulders will thank you.

If You Don't Work Behind a Desk

Not everybody goes to an office every day. An estimated 58 percent of the population works either in retail, manufacturing, or some other occupation that requires mostly standing all day or another body position unrelated to typing and paperwork. (These include dentists, mail carriers, cashiers, deliverypeople, teachers, etc.) It is impossible for me to go through each and every occupation, but there are aspects to standing and lifting for a healthy, comfortable back that apply to all walks of life.

Those who stand for much of the day should keep their torso, head, and neck in line and vertical as much as possible. That helps keep the spinal column aligned in its natural curves. It is also a good idea to elevate one foot on a footrest or footstool for part of the time. That reduces stress in the lower back.

When lifting, use common sense. Handling manual material accounts for up to 40 percent of workers' compensation claims in the United States, but you don't have to be among the statistics. Here are some key points to remember:

- Keep in mind that, on average, a woman's arms and torso can lift 60 percent as much as a man's.
- Remember that strength declines with age to some degree. Your ability to lift and carry at age 65 is about 75 percent of what it was at age 25.
- Don't lift things that are heavier than one third to one half of your body weight. (Sliding, if possible, is less of a challenge to the back than lifting. Push rather than pull when you slide.)
- Lift like a forklift, not a crane. That is, always keep your back straight when you lift. Bend your knees and get closer to the floor if you must. Do not bend at the waist. Bending your knees to pick up a heavy object puts more of the weight on your leg muscles, which are naturally stronger than your back muscles. In addition, keep the load as close to your body as possible, which will keep your back from stretching in ways it shouldn't. As you lift and carry, tighten your abdominal muscles (hold in your stomach). That will support your spine. Keep breathing! If you have to hold your breath to lift something, it is too heavy—you shouldn't be lifting it.
- Wear proper footwear. Wearing heels or otherwise inappro-

priate shoes while lifting something can exacerbate back pain by putting extra pressure on a body that is already off balance and out of alignment. Consider that high heels throw forward all the body's weight as they tip the pelvis out front. This, in turn, contorts the natural curvature of the spine, rendering it much harder to keep upright and thereby forcing a woman to apply a lot more muscular effort to keep from falling forward. That effort comes largely from the lower back, resulting in an unnatural arch that can easily result in back pain.

Mix Up Your Work Environment

I cannot stress enough that whether you sit or stand for most of the day, it is important to change positions regularly so that no one part of your body's scaffolding becomes too taxed. Take frequent breaks, walking around for a few minutes when possible. At your workstation, stretch your fingers, hands, arms, and torso periodically, all of which will relieve pressure on your spine by tensing and then relaxing your muscles. Wiggle your toes, too.

One way that I have mixed up my desk area is that I now use an exercise ball (65 cm, large) as my chair for at least half of the day while I am seated at my desk. The constant movement of the ball keeps my trunk continually engaged while I sit. The best part is that I just can't slouch while I am seated. If I did, I would fall off the ball. I really love it and recommend it highly!

IN BED

I had been married for fifteen years when my husband and I decided it was time to buy a new mattress. The mattress we had been sleeping on was more than twenty years old. Actually, it wasn't one mattress; it was two. They were from twin beds that my college roommate and I had used, and my husband and I had pushed them together to make a king-size bed.

We were *ten years late* in making our purchase. Most health care professionals specializing in sleep and body alignment recommend replacing your mattress every eight to ten years.

Once we did take the plunge and treat ourselves to a decent mattress, we were a bit like the princess (and prince) and the pea. The first one we bought was too soft; we didn't know how to choose one in the store. But the second one, firmer but not ultrafirm, was just right.

Now, my husband and I look forward more to going to bed (yes, you understood that correctly) and also sleep more soundly. The new mattress has helped with my recurring back pain, too.

It's not surprising. When you sleep, the body is compressed by gravity in a different way from when you sit or stand, and the natural shape of the spine still needs to be fully supported.

How Do You Choose a Good Mattress?

It's not all that easy to find the right mattress. Just about all of the mattress studies on record have been conducted by mattress manufacturers, which hardly makes the research arm's-length investigations. (A small, independent study out of Spain a couple of years ago suggests that a medium-firm mattress is best for alleviating low back pain because it provides support without putting undue stress on pressure points.) On top of that, there's an endless array of mattresses—and prices—to choose from. Some range as high as $10,000 and up.

My own gut, and that of a number of orthopedic surgeons, says you can get a decent queen or king mattress and box spring for $1,000 to $2,000—not a lot of money for something you're going to spend seven to eight hours a day on for the next ten years or so. Generally, mattresses in this price range will have a high coil count and thick padding, indications of quality.

Note, however, that coil count and padding thickness alone cannot tell you which mattress to buy. There's no single one that works best for all people and no single one that works best for alleviating back pain. It's a matter of personal preference and comfort. You've got to lie down on some mattresses at the store and see which is best for *you*.

Here are some pointers, however, that may help as you winnow down the options. When you try out a mattress at the store, your shoulders and hips should press into it. At the same time, the mattress should rise up to meet the arch of your back and neck and the curves of your waist and knees, which are more narrow. In other words, your spine should be the same lying down as standing up— in its natural curvature.

Superfirm mattresses might not be able to accomplish this because they don't allow the body to sink in quite enough so that the arch of the back and neck are fully supported. And if a mattress is too soft, it'll be too hammock-like, giving the body too much of a curl.

Lie on each mattress in which you're interested for five to ten minutes. If you sleep with a significant other, lie down with that person to see how the mattress feels with the two of you on it. It feels strange to do that in the middle of a large store, but that's how much time it really takes to decide whether the mattress seems right for you. If my husband and I had known that, we wouldn't have had to replace our first new mattress within a month of buying it.

Never go by terms such as "firm." One company's "firm" may be another manufacturer's "extra-firm" and your "medium." You really have to try it out for yourself. In the same vein, don't be swayed by definitions such as "orthopedic." That's more marketing hype than science.

Taking Care of Your Mattress at Home

Once you buy a mattress and have it delivered, reposition it every six months to ensure that it wears evenly. That means rotating it 180 degrees and flipping it. Once the mattress begins to sag in the middle, or if you're simply no longer comfortable on it, it's time for a new one.

Pillow Talk

As with a mattress, the choice of pillow is a matter of personal preference. While pillows in general help provide support for the head, neck, and shoulders and also keep them in alignment, there's no one right pillow that does that equally well for all people. If you prefer a relatively puffy pillow, use that kind. If you like your pillow flat, that's okay, too. Do keep in mind that pillow firmness fades over time. Replace as you see fit.

Sleeping Position

Sleep time is really the only time that the muscles and ligaments in your spine can completely relax—a necessary component for healing an aching back. Contrary to popular belief, there is no one right position to sleep in—a good thing since it's hard to exert control over the position in which you fall asleep and *stay* asleep.

Having said that, if you sleep on your back, try keeping a small pillow tucked underneath the backs of your knees. That completely unloads spinal stress—a good thing if you suffer from lower back pain. If you sleep on your side, you might want to put a pillow *between* your knees. That helps keep pressure off the hips and lumbar region (particularly useful for those who have pain from osteo-arthritis or spinal stenosis, and tend to curl up their knees into the fetal position). And if you sleep on your stomach, try placing a flat pillow beneath your stomach and hips. That, too, can relieve stress on the hips and lower spine (and is said to work especially well for relieving pain from degenerative disc disease).

EVERYDAY ERGONOMICS— AT HOME AND ELSEWHERE

In the scheme of things, it's relatively easy to make sure that the ergonomics of your workplace and your bedroom are right for you. You're pretty much the only one who uses them, and your roles in those two places are pretty much the same from day to day. But what about the ergonomics of the other third of your life—during which you're awake but not earning your salary? How do you make sure your environment is suited to your back then?

The aim is to apply the principles from your workday life to your life outside of your job. Take your car, for instance. Some people spend upwards of two hours a day in their autos, depending on their commute. If they're real estate agents, truck drivers, or people who make sales calls, their wheels *are* their offices. The aim in a car seat is the same as in a desk chair. The back, the lower back in particular, should be fully supported by the seat. Some people may have to put a rolled-up towel behind them to get the lower back support they need.

And just as with a computer desk, you should not have to lean forward to reach the steering wheel and other controls. They should be within arm's reach as you sit comfortably.

At home, chairs you sit in for any length of time should also support your back. I know someone with a lovely Shaker-style rocker that she very much admired, but, frustratingly, it was too big for her to use comfortably. She could not sit back in it because her feet would not touch the floor, and that meant that whenever she did use it, her back was not getting any support from the chair back. The solution, which she wished she had realized sooner, was simple. She found a matching Shaker footrest, which enabled her to rest her feet flatly while sitting back in the chair and getting her spine in alignment.

You should also make it as easy as possible at home to bend, reach, and lift things. Think of your kitchen. A lot of people keep things they rarely use on high shelves that are difficult to reach. If it's something heavy and bulky, like a large, delicate platter or piece of baking machinery, it could be very awkward to get it down. *Never* twist, turn, or stretch as you're lifting—these movements can easily throw out your back. If the step stool is too far away, move it down so that you can retrieve the item without straining. If no amount of step stool maneuvering will allow you to reach for something comfortably on a high shelf, ask someone else to do it. The couple of minutes you might save in doing it yourself by contorting your body can cause you weeks of back or neck pain.

It's the same with laundry, gardening supplies, groceries, and anything else that requires back muscle. Never lift more than you comfortably can; make two trips. Keep often-used items within easy reach. If the item is very heavy, slide it if possible. And keep your back straight as often as you can. Don't bend over at the waist to pick up weeds; bend at the knees. Don't bend over at the waist to get clothes out of a front-facing dryer. Bring over a step stool to reach bedding on a high shelf that you haven't used all season; and so on.

I urge you to set aside some time to assess your environment and take any (and all) necessary steps to bring it into ergonomic compliance with your body. Sometimes a few small changes can make all the difference. Certainly, without this care you are giving your back short shrift and minimizing the benefits of any other back-healthy steps you take.

PART 3

When to Seek
Professional Help

CHAPTER 7

A Team of Strong Back Experts: Your Primary Care Physician and Beyond

◈

I've had issues with my neck and my back for close to ten years. When there's a flare-up, it's like knifing pain if I try to turn more than 5 degrees. What I've done for relief through the years is go to a chiropractor—three to five appointments over about a month's time. The pain melts over the course of each session. You can feel a release, and then it kind of just melts away, like someone injected Percocet into my arteries. People have said to me, 'Chiropractors, they're quacks.' But a chiropractor, for me—I would swear by it.

—CHRISTINA

O bviously, if you get recurrent back pain or an episode of back pain that just won't quit, you're going to want to see your primary care physician to get to the bottom of the problem. But there are other types of health professionals who might be able to help ease your back pain, too. A number of them were mentioned in the chapter on stress: psychologists, massage therapists, and yoga and tai chi instructors, for instance.

There are also several other types of health care providers who may be able to do something for a problem back, including physicians with varying specialties. For instance, a *physiatrist* is an M.D. who focuses specifically on physical and rehabilitation medicine, which means she or he utilizes a number of conservative treatments for optimal function of the musculoskeletal system. These include therapeutic exercise, heat and cold therapy, biofeedback, medications (including injections), and physical therapy. (Sometimes a physiatrist leads a team of specialists in these areas to help patients.) A physiatrist will also do a lifestyle assessment with you to set goals and also help avoid pain recurrence. And she or he will continually measure your progress while counseling/educating you about techniques for self-management of your pain. In short, a physiatrist helps you reverse functional losses and improve quality of life without resorting to surgery. (To become a board-certified physiatrist, a physician must pass a written and oral examination administered by the American Board of Physical and Rehabilitation Medicine.)

Osteopaths are physicians with the letters D.O. after their name rather than M.D. They complete four years of osteopathic medical school and are licensed to prescribe medications, but they also receive an additional 300 to 500 hours in the study of hands-on manual medicine and the body's musculoskeletal system. Somewhat like a chiropractor, an osteopath often uses a treatment called manipulation, gently applying a precise amount of force to promote healthy movement of tissues, eliminate abnormal movements, and relieve compressed bones and joints. Like M.D.s, osteopaths can be primary care providers themselves, physiatrists, surgeons, etc.

Other types of physicians who may be of help include *neurologists,* who can treat back pain related to damaged or irritated nerves, and *orthopedic surgeons,* who are sometimes called upon for consultations regarding such things as damaged vertebrae and, when necessary, surgery.

Along with these different kinds of physicians and the specialists I mentioned in the chapter on stress, there are three other types of health care providers who may be able to do something for a problem back: *physical and occupational therapists, chiropractors,* and *acupuncturists.* What follows is a rundown on each of them, including their benefits and limitations.

PHYSICAL THERAPISTS

I am a big fan of physical therapists. When I was training for the Boston Marathon a couple of years ago, physical therapy helped me get over a foot injury that was threatening to get in the way of my completing the race.

As far as back pain, physical therapy can be so effective that it is sometimes a way to avoid back surgery. It is normally recommended for back pain that persists for longer than two weeks.

Teaching You to Be Your Own Physical Therapist

The best thing about physical therapists is that much of what they do is show you how to become your own therapist. That is, after they help you get better, they teach ways for you to heal *yourself* as you go about your daily routine instead of making a new injury worse or causing reinjury. Some of those ways are considered "passive" because they are done to you; others are "active" because you carry them out yourself.

Passive Physical Therapy Treatments

There are four types of passive physical therapy treatments.

1. *Heat or ice packs.* Both heat and ice help reduce muscle spasms and inflammation. Working with a physical therapist, you'll find out which works better for you. Sometimes the two are alternated. Most useful during the first few days after a back injury, the ice or heat tends to be applied for ten to twenty minutes every couple of hours. (Heat tends not to be applied within the first forty-eight hours.)

2. *Lontophoresis.* This is the treatment I underwent for my foot injury. It involves delivering steroids to a part of the body that is causing pain. The steroids provide an anti-inflammatory effect. The way it works is that steroids are applied right to the skin, after which an electrical current is used that allows the steroids to migrate under the skin to the injured spot.

3. *TENS units.* With this form of physical therapy, a transcutaneous electrical nerve stimulator (TENS) unit transmits low-voltage electrical stimulation through the skin (via electrodes) to override pain signals normally recognized by the brain. If the patient experiences substantial relief, she may be given a TENS unit to be used at home for long-term back pain relief.

4. *Ultrasound.* Ultrasound can be particularly helpful when it comes to relieving acute episodes of lower back pain. It may

even promote tissue healing. It's a form of deep heating. Sound waves are applied right to the skin and from there penetrate soft tissues to get to the root of the pain.

Active Physical Therapy Treatments

Active physical therapy for back pain generally consists of an exercise program tailored specifically to you—your pain, your lifestyle, and your injury. A physical therapist will show you pain-relieving stretches and also devise a resistance (strength-training) program specifically targeted to your particular back problem. Low-impact aerobic conditioning will probably be included as well. Just as I recommend in chapter 4, a physical therapist will usually encourage you to walk, bike, or swim several times a week.

Along with encouraging various exercises, a physical therapist will work to limit back pain by advising you on proper body posture and body motion in your daily chores, both at work and at home. That way, you'll be using your body to advantage rather than disadvantage, increasing your physical functioning and range of motion all the while—and reducing your risk for back injury in the future.

Finding a Competent Physical Therapist

Finding a qualified physical therapist is easy. Physical therapists are licensed via the American Physical Therapy Association (see Resources). If your physician refers you to a physical therapist, there's a reasonable chance your health insurance will pay for a set number of visits.

CHIROPRACTORS

Despite the fact that chiropractors constitute the third largest group of health care professionals in the United States (after physicians and

What About *Occupational* Therapists?

While a physical therapist will help you get past an injury, an occupational therapist works on getting people with an injury or disability better able to function in their daily lives. They focus on *context.* For instance, for someone with a back injury, an occupational therapist might perform a comprehensive evaluation of both the job site and the home and then make recommendations about how to adapt routines so that what was difficult or impossible to do becomes doable. They might even recommend various pieces of equipment to improve independent functioning.

Occupational therapists also give guidance to family members and caregivers for helping a person deal with activities of daily living, focusing on the social and emotional effects of illness and injury as well as the physiological ones. Occupational therapists, who must complete clinical internships in a variety of health care settings *and* pass a national exam, often work with people who have work-related lower back problems as well as those with spinal cord injuries. (See Resources for more information on occupational therapists.)

dentists), and despite the fact that their services are partially covered by Medicare, there is probably more disagreement about their value than about the value of any other type of health care professional. Some people, like Christina quoted at the beginning of this chapter, swear by chiropractors, saying they alleviate nagging back pain quickly and painlessly. Others say their diplomas are not worth the paper they're printed on. I don't agree with that line of thinking. But part of the reason for such divergent views stems, no doubt, from chiropractic's origins, along with the belief of some chiropractors that they can heal conditions that have nothing to do with a bad back.

A Quick History of Chiropractic Medicine

In 1895, a grocer in Iowa named Daniel David Palmer was said to have cured a man's deafness by pushing on one of the vertebrae in his back. Palmer, considered a "healer," also worked to combine the mending of broken bones with a restored flow of energy that would supposedly right all kinds of wrongs in the body, not just those leading to back pain. It was his belief that interference with the flow of good energy through the nerves and spine caused disease and that, via spinal manipulation, the energy could be freed up and the body could heal itself.

Out of that theory and approach the profession of chiropractic grew. (The word chiropractic literally means "done by hand.") In early chiropractic education, future practitioners were taught that "vertebral subluxations"—pinched nerves or other abnormalities in the spine—were responsible for everything from bronchitis to kidney disease to constipation. Adjust the right bone in the spine, and health in another area would be restored.

The theory has no scientific backing. In fact, the idea of subluxations wreaking havoc with your body is often played down in chiropractic education these days, with the emphasis more squarely on neuromusculoskeletal problems that directly affect the back. Still, the subluxation theory continues to be at least part of the education at all seventeen chiropractic colleges in the United States. At the very least, it gets covered under chiropractic philosophy or chiropractic theory.

Chiropractors who subscribe closely to the subluxation theory and tell you they can do much more for you than alleviate back pain are the ones who legitimize any charges of quackery. Those who limit their practices to treating real spine or joint problems, on the other hand, might really be able to help where another health care professional has hit a dead end in working to minimize your pain.

How a Chiropractor Can Help

There's no question that a chiropractor can often alleviate back pain or spasms by "unlocking" a stiff joint or muscle. Specifically, she or he engages in spinal manipulation by applying high-velocity arm thrusts (or pressure from mechanical devices) to a vertebra in the area of the spine that is causing the problem. As a result, pressure is released in the problem area (it's sometimes referred to as the popping treatment), and pain subsides.

For neck pain, the evidence is mixed, at best. Some studies do suggest that manipulation brings relief, and Christina, the woman quoted at the beginning of this chapter, would certainly agree. But in the main, there's no evidence that chiropractic thrusts meant to ease neck discomfort are any more effective than treatment with such things as massage or hot and cold packs.

Choosing the Right Chiropractor

If you have back pain that you haven't been able to alleviate, by all means a decision to see a chiropractor can be a reasonable one. But first see your physician to make sure your pain doesn't have a serious underlying cause like a fracture or perhaps even a tumor. Chiropractors are appropriate health care choices for certain types of back pain, but not pain with evidence of nerve problems or major trauma.

Once you do make the decision to see a chiropractor, make sure she or he deals only with spinal problems. Problems unrelated to the spine cannot be corrected with spinal "fixes." Also, steer clear of any chiropractor who:

- Recommends particular diets or nutritional supplements and perhaps even sells them. Chiropractors are not trained to dispense nutrition advice. Moreover, *any* doctor who sells you a remedy he recommends has a direct conflict of interest that should be seen as a major red flag.
- Advises against immunizations. Some chiropractors believe, incorrectly, that as long as your spine is healthy, your natural defenses will be able to fight off infections. Not true.
- Voices mistrust of physicians, perhaps by refusing to refer you to one. The community of medical doctors is not out to "get you" or cheat you. A chiropractor who suggests they are is not to be trusted.
- Says you should come in for spinal manipulations periodically, whether you feel well or not. A chiropractor can only alleviate pain that's already there. There's no such thing as preventive spinal manipulation.

Try searching for a competent chiropractor through the American Chiropractic Association. That organization endorses the use of chiropractic only for the treatment of musculoskeletal problems and not for conditions in other parts of the body.

Note that common reactions to chiropractic manipulation are aching and soreness in the spine, lasting no longer than twenty-four hours and generally only a few hours. If overall relief from back pain is not achieved after several sessions over a few weeks, chiropractic manipulation of your spine is probably not the answer to your problem.

ACUPUNCTURISTS

If chiropractic seems outside the boundaries of mainstream medicine, acupuncture is even more so, despite the fact that it has been practiced in Asia for more than 2,500 years. Consider the Eastern philosophy behind it. Essentially, the theory is that illness takes hold when someone is out of balance with nature and its two opposing forces: yin, which is the passive, feminine force, and yang, which stands for aggressive, masculine qualities.

Acupuncture is said to restore balance via the insertion of fine needles at various points on fourteen meridians, or pathways, that are mapped on the human body. It's through those meridians that flows one's life force, or qi (pronounced "chee"). And by placing needles at any of some 2,000 points along the meridians, interruptions or bottlenecking of qi can be smoothed away, allowing for the resumption of a healthy flow of energy.

If it sounds kooky, that's because by the standards of Western medicine, it is. There is no biologically proven basis for showing evidence of the existence of meridians, let alone "life force." But by the same token, there is a limit to what Western medicine can measure, and there are millennia of anecdotal evidence to believe the ancient healers were onto something very helpful.

Better still, scientists *have* been able to uncover scientific possibilities for why acupuncture appears to be able to reduce pain in some instances—which helps explain why at least 15 million Americans have undergone acupuncture treatment.

Clues to Acupuncture's Potential Effectiveness

The turning point for acupuncture's image came in the late 1990s. A panel of a dozen scientists convened by the National Institutes of Health reached consensus, via research they evaluated, that inserting needles into the skin apparently stimulates the release of endorphins and other opiods, chemicals in the body that act as natural pain relievers. Other research has shown that acupuncture causes changes in the secretions of hormones and other compounds in the brain like serotonin, which can influence someone's perception of pain.

It may even be that acupuncture changes the flow of blood through the body. Some of the focus at the National Institutes of Health conference was on research that used single proton emission computed tomography, a procedure by which blood flow can be measured in the brain. What was found was that after acupuncture sessions in people experiencing pain, a region of the brain called the thalamus "lit up," which meant there was a surge in the flow of blood

It Doesn't Hurt

It might seem as though the insertion of acupuncture needles on different parts of the body would hurt. It doesn't. The Food and Drug Administration–approved needles are hair-thin—about twenty times thinner than a typical needle used for injections.

The needles, up to about twenty in a single session, are often left in place for fifteen to thirty minutes. Some practitioners insert needles and then turn them in one direction or the other, depending on the desired effect. In such cases, a needle may be left in for only ten seconds or so, then removed and inserted in a different spot in the same patient.

there. That's important because prior to the subjects' acupuncture, blood flow in the thalamus was sub-par.

By the end of the conference, the National Institutes of Health panel said that the 200-plus studies they looked over suggested that acupuncture helps relieve nausea and vomiting after an operation; pain following dental procedures; and nausea and vomiting after chemotherapy.

There were also a number of conditions listed for which the evidence was not as convincing but intriguing nonetheless. These included detox from drugs and alcohol, stroke rehabilitation, headaches, menstrual cramps, tennis elbow, general muscle pain, osteoarthritis, carpal tunnel syndrome, asthma, and, yes, lower back pain. Future research will shed more light on the usefulness of acupuncture for back pain and other medical problems.

To be sure, even the best research on acupuncture has some hard-to-overcome limitations that make assessing its benefits difficult. For instance, it can be hard to tell whether the acupuncture itself is doing something, or whether there's a strong placebo effect at work. After all, acupuncturists, unlike physicians, who are increasingly under the time constraints of managed care, often spend a lot of time talking with their patients—up to forty-five minutes or an hour. They also tend to do their work in a soothing and relaxing environment, unlike a white, sterile doctor's office. Those differences in themselves might affect a person's perceptions of the helpfulness of the treatment.

Then, too, it's not easy to judge pain levels objectively. It's not the same as, say, checking someone's blood pressure before and after she takes a blood pressure drug. Where one person perceives a diminishment of pain, another might perceive no difference at all.

For all of that, however, someone who has exhausted other avenues of relief from back pain to little or no effect might want to give acupuncture a try. After all, less pain, even without knowledge of the *reason* for less pain, is very desirable.

Note that acupuncture is not totally risk-free. In rare cases, needles inserted an inch deep have rendered people vulnerable to nerve and tissue damage and other complications.

Note, too, that few health insurers cover acupuncture sessions, and prices run from at least $40 to $100 per session, with most acupuncturists recommending at least a few sessions. In addition, there is no mandatory standard of training or credentialing. Acupuncture schooling varies considerably from state to state.

If you do decide to try acupuncture for back pain, adhere to the following guidelines.

1. Make sure you get examined by a physician first to rule out causes of back pain that an acupuncturist would not be able to treat. Going to a health care professional who cannot help you wastes time, prolongs pain, and perhaps worsens a condition—rather than alleviates it. You should also talk to your primary health care provider about seeing an acupuncturist if you have a pacemaker, a bleeding disorder, infections of the skin or skin disease, or are pregnant.

2. Find out which school the acupuncturist was trained at. Then find out whether the school is accredited by the Accreditation Commission for Acupuncture and Oriental medicine (ACAOM), which is based in Silver Spring, Maryland. ACAOM's accreditation process is recognized by the U.S. Department of Education.

3. Allow for healthy skepticism. For instance, many acupuncturists use herbs and other remedies in addition to needles. But the research on herbs is spotty, as are rules governing

their sale and manufacture. You don't want your treatment based on one person's "sense" of what's a good idea.

4. Be certain that the acupuncturist uses disposable needles. Cases of hepatitis B have resulted from careless needle handling.

THE CHOICE IS YOURS

With this chapter, I am not trying to push you into seeing a health care provider you may not feel comfortable with. But I do think it is important to know that the options for getting back pain under control are more numerous than many people realize. Christina, the woman mentioned at the beginning of this chapter, is a highly educated professional and by looks and demeanor is not the sort of person you'd automatically assume would seek out someone other than her physician. But as she observes, "if something like chiropractic is covered by almost every health care plan, I wouldn't put it in the category of 'alternative' medicine."

CHAPTER 8

Do You Need Back Surgery?

I had had some back pain as a teenager, after lifting a heavy pa-
tient in a nursing home during a summer job before my senior
year of high school. But with exercises and anti-inflammatory
drugs, it went away. Then, when I was 36, the pain came back,
and it was excruciating. Like a knife. It went from my back all the
way down my left leg. I was numb from my knee on down and
was walking with a limp. I literally had to pick up my foot to take
a step. I couldn't lie down, sit, or stand; I couldn't get into a com-
fortable position.

I went to see an orthopedic surgeon, who thought I had a her-
niated disc. A CT scan confirmed his diagnosis. At first he put me
on some meds—an anti-inflammatory drug, plus a steroid. But
after a month—and that included physical therapy, too—it hadn't
gotten any better. I'm a hairdresser and was limping around the
beauty parlor in pain. The doctor told me to consider surgery.

I told him to do it. I had three young children—12, 10, and 7.
I wanted to Rollerblade with them. I wanted to play with them. I

told him that if he couldn't get me out of pain, he might as well put me in a nursing home.

They took out 40 percent of my disc. The relief after surgery was immediate.

—RHONDA

R honda is one of the extremely lucky ones. An estimated 400,000 back surgeries are performed each year in the United States. But the unfortunate truth is that *fewer than 5 percent of them are believed to be effective in significantly reducing back pain.* And FBSS—failed back surgery syndrome—is all too common. Frequently, people end up in worse pain after the surgery than before.

Why such a gap between the number of back surgeries performed and the number of people the operations help?

One reason is that a lot of people opt for surgery as a last resort, when everything else has failed. They are desperate. But surgery is not the automatic route to go just because pain persists despite all previous efforts to dispel it. Sometimes the answer is to learn ways to manage or cope with the pain, get it in the background, rather than try to cut it away. Consider that among the most common causes of back pain are problems such as muscle strains, which simply cannot be mechanically corrected through surgery.

Another issue is that diagnoses of back problems that precipitate surgery can be very misleading. Doctors can't even conclusively diagnose the reason for the pain in many cases. Let's say, for instance, that someone has been suffering lower back pain for months and finally goes for an MRI (magnetic resonance imaging) or a CT scan to check for degenerated, bulging, or herniated discs. Compromised discs will frequently be found, and they can be repaired or removed through surgery. But they're often *not* the cause of the pain. The fact is that a lot of people have misshapen discs that they have been living with for years, decades even, without the disc degeneration causing a whit of discomfort. In one study, researchers performed MRIs on people who had no back pain whatsoever yet found that more than half of them had bulging discs nonetheless. The bottom line: Only sometimes do mechanical problems such as damaged discs correlate with pain.

Even when a disc does cause pain, say, as a result of some kind of structural problem that makes it press on nerves, it often resolves on its own. With proper care and sometimes just with time, it can make a subtle shift that provides total or near total relief. In other words, what seems like a need for surgery could just be a need to wait out the pain a little.

The level of pain is not an indicator for surgery, either. Even very debilitating pain that lasts for months often resolves, especially with appropriate lifestyle steps. In a study conducted several years ago at the Physicians Neck and Back Clinic in Minnesota, thirty-eight patients whose doctors had recommended back surgery agreed to participate in a ten-week program, during which they engaged in an aggressive regimen of strengthening exercises. In the end, only three of the original thirty-eight elected to undergo the surgery—presumably, most were feeling better enough not to go under the knife, after all. It would seem to indicate that lifestyle avenues often remain insufficiently explored.

Finally, factors outside of damage to the back influence the success or failure of back surgery. Research has found that people with back problems who are depressed or subject to anxiety or social difficulties or lead less than healthful lives—smoking, remaining sedentary, eating poorly, and so on—are less apt to benefit from back surgery than others. Why? Pain is tricky and often hard to pin down, with input from the whole body and the whole lifestyle. Thus, surgically fixing a herniated disc or a narrowed spinal canal doesn't automatically make everything right; there's a holistic aspect to back pain that often requires a holistic approach.

ARE YOU A GOOD CANDIDATE FOR BACK SURGERY?

Despite the fact that so few people with back pain have anything to gain by putting themselves through the rigor of an operation and its aftermath of slow rehabilitation, there are some who *can* benefit—as long as they realize that surgery rarely causes the pain to subside completely, and as long as they recognize that sometimes the relief is temporary, perhaps lasting just a few years.

How do you begin to consider whether surgery might be right for you?

Certainly, you should first give every lifestyle step recommended in this book, in conjunction with recommendations by your doctor, your very best shot. They are very powerful interventions, even though they are not technologically complicated.

If pain persists over at least a month—or gets worse—despite your taking appropriate lifestyle measures, it's worth thinking about going for a diagnostic workup. You should also go for a workup if:

- You have pain radiating from your backside down your leg, often accompanied by numbness or tingling, or severe leg weakness. These can be signs of sciatica, which is pressure on a nerve that runs out of the spinal column and down the leg, and they can also signal a severely herniated disc or spinal tumor. Pain arising from all of these conditions can potentially be helped with surgery.

- Your pain was caused by an accident or you have a high risk for osteoporosis. You may have fractured a vertebra, or bone, in your spine.
- You are experiencing loss of bladder or bowel control or weight loss that has nothing to do with dieting. Coupled with back pain, these can be signs of spinal cancer or other serious problems and necessitate an immediate visit to your physician.

Diagnostic Tools

All patients who might be candidates for back surgery should start by undergoing a thorough check in the doctor's office during which a careful history is taken and a physical examination conducted. Often, this measure alone is enough to rule out surgery or indicate further testing—imaging—to help determine whether surgery is in fact warranted.

If imaging is called for, X-rays are one way to go. But they're not highly sensitive on their own for detecting causes of back pain. Also, back X-rays expose patients to many times the radiation of a chest X-ray or mammogram—they are not totally benign.

Many patients will end up getting a CT scan or MRI. Not only are they better at detecting early spinal infections and cancers, they also are good for identifying herniated discs and spinal stenosis—narrowing of the spinal canal that can cause painful pressure on nerve roots. X-rays cannot detect these conditions because they cannot "see" the soft tissue involved.

Of course, since problem discs and stenosis don't necessarily lead

Surgery May Be Right For

- Herniated or degenerated disc
- Spinal fracture
- Spinal cancer
- Spinal stenosis (narrowing of the spinal column)
- Cauda equina syndrome (damage to nerve roots)
- Severe cases of spinal infection
- Severe scoliosis (curvature of the spine)
- Kyphosis (a humpback deformity)
- Spondylolisthesis (forward slippage of a segment of the spine)

to back pain, the specialist looking over the images has to make a determination about whether the anatomical abnormality present could be pressing on a nerve in a way that is causing the discomfort.

Other diagnostic tools that may be used are myelograms, which are X-rays combined with a special dye injected into the spinal sac to highlight the spinal cord and nerves; electromyograms and nerve conduction studies, which look at how nerves and muscles work together (testing, specifically, for whether impulses from the brain or spinal cord are blocked); and discography, an injection into a disc(s) that tries to determine whether there is any damage and whether it is causing pain.

If Surgery is Recommended

Keep in mind that surgery for back pain is almost always elective. You make the decision *with* the doctor, rather than passively follow her or his advice. That means you need to understand to what degree the doctor thinks the operation will improve your pain. (A 30 to 50 percent improvement is considered very good.) You also need to fully understand the risks. Make sure the doctor explains what could go wrong when operating by the spinal column.

Other things to discuss with the physician are whether there are alternatives to the surgery; whether the condition is likely to worsen without the operation; and what's involved in recovery and rehabilitation.

No matter how comfortable you are with the specialist who talks with you about surgery, *be sure to get a second opinion.* I cannot stress this enough. Back surgery is simply too big an undertaking to proceed without two medical opinions.

Types of Back Surgery

There are several types of back operations, each of which works to correct different problems. More are being developed all the time; it's an evolving science.

Discectomy

This type of surgery involves the removal of herniated disc material that is pressing on a nerve root or the spinal cord itself. Sometimes the surgeon removes disc *fragments* that are protruding into the spinal canal. Most patients stay in the hospital one to two nights, although day surgery for discectomy is not unheard of.

In uncomplicated cases, the likelihood of good to excellent relief of pain, including relief of leg pain that occurs as a result of a pinched nerve, is pretty high. Numbness may persist for a while, however.

A variation on discectomy is *percutaneous discectomy.* In this type of surgery, which is sometimes recommended for sciatica or scoliosis as well as for cauda equina syndrome, the surgeon isn't looking directly at the compressed root. Instead, the procedure uses continuous X-ray monitoring, or fluoroscopy, which allows for tracking movement in the body. Specifically, X-rays are directed at the spine, and the pictures that are taken are displayed on a TV-like monitor in the operating room, allowing the doctor to see where she or he is working.

The advantages of percutaneous discectomy are that it takes only about an hour (often in a surgery center), generally requires a bandage over the (small) point of incision rather than stitches, and generates only mild postoperative pain. Unfortunately, it is less effective than traditional discectomy. Without a direct view of the compressed root, there's less of a chance that pressure, and pain, will be reduced.

A second variation on discectomy is *microdiscectomy*. It's similar to a percutaneous discectomy in that the compressed root is not viewed directly. Instead, the surgeon uses a microscope or other magnifying instrument to look at the affected disc and nerves and then removes any herniated material, also through a small incision in the back.

Laminectomy

A laminectomy is often performed to relieve stenosis—narrowing of the spinal column that can cause not only back pain but also leg pain. Generally conducted on the lower back, it involves literally removing the back side of the spinal canal, or lamina, to relieve pressure on roots. The surgeon makes a small incision in the lower back, then pushes aside fat and muscle to expose the spine itself. The procedure then often involves removing protruding bone in the form of a bone spur. There might also be removal of a herniated disc that's pressing on a nerve, which means a laminectomy and a discectomy are performed during the same operation. (That was the case in

Rhonda's situation, mentioned at the start of this chapter.) Ligaments that are pressing on a nerve may be removed, too.

Spinal Fusion
Spinal fusion is a more involved surgery than laminectomy. It involves joining two bones, or vertebrae, to make one, and thereby stabilizes the back in a spot that the movement of two bones is causing pain. (When you break your arm, a plaster cast essentially allows two bones to become one.)

Traditionally, spinal fusions were used to correct spondylolisthesis—forward slippage of the spine. But they are now used to cor-

New Spinal Fusion Alternative

In 2004, the U.S. Government approved the use of an artificial disc for treating pain associated with degenerative disc disease. Meant to replace a diseased or damaged disc, it is intended for people who have degenerative disc disease in the lumbar spine and have experienced no relief from low back pain after at least six months of nonsurgical treatment.

The disc itself is made of plastic that is sandwiched between two pieces of metal. During an operation, the diseased or damaged disc is removed and the new, synthetic one placed in the spine through a small incision just below the belly button. This helps restore movement, just like a spinal fusion is meant to do.

There are still kinks to be worked out. Sometimes too much movement is restored, overstressing the device. Sometimes not enough movement is restored. Long-term safety and effectiveness also remain unknown. But it is a step in the right direction away from very involved spinal fusions.

rect a number of other deformities as well as improve stability after, say, a fracture.

During the operation, small pieces of bone are needed from else-where to fuse the two bones at issue. The extra bone used for the grafting typically comes from somewhere else in the body—often the hip or pelvis. Apparatus such as screws, plates, rods, and cages is then put in place to facilitate the fusion (just as a plaster cast on the arm facilitates fusion), which takes about three months. (The screws generally remain in the back for life.)

I want to stress here that while spinal fusions can definitely be called for in cases of fracture and spinal cancer, their track record for relieving lower back pain is mixed. In a Scandinavian study, only about 15 percent of people who underwent the operation to relieve pain in the lumbar spine ended up with an "excellent" result two years out. Really know what you're getting into before undergoing a fusion. Sometimes a less complicated operation can be used to treat the same kind of pain.

Vertebroplasty/Kyphoplasty

These procedures, both relatively new in the arsenal of back inter-ventions, are used for people who suffer compression fractures of the vertebrae. Such fractures often result from osteoporosis, although cancer such as multiple myeloma can also be a cause. A vertebra be-comes so weak that it compresses, sometimes to the point of ending up only half its original thickness. That causes misalignment of the spine, which, of course, can lead to pain.

Vertebroplasty, which has the benefit of not being a very invasive procedure, involves injecting "cement" directly into fractured bone, thereby shoring it up. The cement hardens, literally, in hours, acting as a sealant and a stabilizer and relieving pain—quickly.

Kyphoplasty is an offshoot of vertebroplasty. It involves using a balloon-like device to bring a vertebra back to its original height and thereby help reverse humpback deformity. That creates a space that gets filled with bone cement to support the bone.

It should be noted that questions have arisen about the effectiveness of both of these procedures. Some patients swear by them; others say their pain did not improve—or worsened. Unfortunately, there are too few clinical trials at this point to come down one way or the other. A thorough discussion with your doctor about the potential pros and cons is definitely in order.

Spinal Cord Stimulation

This newish procedure is not an operation per se but, rather, a form of therapy involving an electric generator that delivers pulses to a specific area of the spinal cord in order to interrupt pain signals. It is often used on people with failed back surgery syndrome.

The way it works is that leads that contain electrodes are implanted, often by laminectomy. An electric current is then delivered via the generator straight to those leads, which are placed near the part of the spinal cord thought to be causing the pain. The number of leads varies, in part due to the specific nerve roots involved and in part due to the level of the patient's pain.

The exact mechanism by which the procedure reduces pain is not yet understood. It seems to be better for alleviating long-term pain than for alleviating an acute bout of pain.

Fluoroscopically Guided Epidural Steroid Injections

This is also not an operation but has the potential to relieve pain caused by irritated spinal nerves. That, in turn, allows a person to continue with, say, her rehabilitation program, to become more comfortable without need of more help, or to remain free of acute pain until her back problem is treated more aggressively. Sometimes the more aggressive treatment involves treating a herniated disc; spinal nerves often become irritated and swollen when they have to move across a damaged disc.

During the thirty-minute injection procedure, both an anesthetic and corticosteroids (anti-inflammatory drugs) are injected into the epidural space around the roots of spinal nerves. The epidural space is sort of like a sleeve that nerves must go through before traveling from the spine into the arms, trunk, and legs. Once in that space (the doctor knows just where to put the injection because of fluoroscopy), the steroids reduce inflammation of affected nerves. Pain is reduced in five to ten days (with the pain becoming worse in some cases before it gets better).

The big caveat is that the procedure works for only about one in two people. For some people, pain is reduced about 30 percent, and they can try another round in hopes of improving the results. (If relief is less than 30 percent, consideration should be given to other avenues of pain relief.)

There are also potential risks, as with any clinical procedure, although they are very uncommon. These include infections, bleeding, and, in extremely rare cases, nerve damage.

MAKING THE CHOICE

In the end, after consultation with your primary care physician and at least two specialists, the choice of whether to undergo back surgery or another back-related procedure is up to you. Keep in mind that if you want an operation and have to go from doctor to doctor before finding one who is willing to perform it, chances are the surgery will not relieve your back pain—and may even increase it. On the other hand, if at least two specialists corroborate in the opinion that surgery will bring relief, *and* if you have realistic expectations that the operation will reduce but probably not eliminate pain, *and* if you're willing to make every effort to continue to support your back through lifestyle measures that include regular exercise and proper ergonomics, surgery might be the right call.

Rhonda knows very well that surgery was a help but not a cure. "I'm not pain free," she says, "and was told I probably wouldn't ever be. I still get backaches in the middle of the night sometimes that wake me up. And occasionally I have to get out of bed carefully. There's a certain vulnerability in my back now. If I'm bending over to pick up a comb I may have dropped, I may get a sharp pain if I bend over the wrong way. And while I went back to most of my previous sports, I did not go back to waterskiing, which I used to do. I'm afraid if I get pulled out of the water the wrong way or lean out of the water the wrong way, I'll hurt my back.

"I also have to exercise regularly. If I take more than one day off, my back starts bothering me.

"But all of this is nothing I can't live with. Life's too short. I'm not the type of person who feels sorry for herself. I even go out dancing sometimes and don't worry about it if I have a little ache and pain the next day."

In other words, Rhonda doesn't just have realistic expectations and an active lifestyle, both of which are necessary for successful surgery. She also has a good outlook on life—crucial for optimal benefits.

Resources

◆

This book provides everything you need to engage in a comprehensive program for preventing or ameliorating back pain and for making your back stronger and healthier in the process. For those who want even more in-depth information on particular topics raised or on finding a specialist in your area to suit particular needs, I have included numerous resources below. Following, you will find organizations, books, Web sites, and more. Keep in mind that Web sites have a way of coming and going—often appearing under new URLs. The sites listed were current at the time I compiled this section. If any are inoperative when you are trying to find them, I encourage you to use a reliable search engine to see if the source can be located at a new site.

Dr. Nelson's Web Site and Books

www.strongwomen.com has a free electronic newsletter, animated exercise programs, and other useful information regarding nutrition and exercise.

Strong Women Stay Young. Rev. ed. Miriam E. Nelson, Ph.D., with Sarah Wernick, Ph.D. (New York: Bantam Books, 2000).

Strong Women Stay Slim. Miriam E. Nelson, Ph.D., with Sarah Wernick, Ph.D. (New York: Bantam Books, 1998).

Strong Women, Strong Bones. Miriam E. Nelson, Ph.D., with Sarah Wernick, Ph.D. (New York: Putnam, 2000).

Strong Women Eat Well. Miriam E. Nelson, Ph.D., with Judy Knipe (New York: Putnam, 2001).

Strong Women and Men *Beat Arthritis.* Miriam E. Nelson, Ph.D., Kristin Baker, Ph.D., and Ronenn Roubenoff, M.D., M.S.H., with Lawrence Lindner, M.A. (New York: Putnam, 2002).

The Strong Women's Journal. Miriam E. Nelson, Ph.D. (New York: Perigee, 2003).

Strong Women, Strong Hearts. Miriam E. Nelson, Ph.D. and Alice Lichtenstein, Ph.D., with Lawrence Lindner, M.A. (New York: Putnam, 2005).

Tufts University Resources

The John Hancock Center for Physical Activity and Nutrition at The Friedman School of Nutrition Science and Policy, Tufts University, maintains a Web site with useful information regarding ongoing research and programs such as the community-based StrongWomen Program. www.go.tufts.edu/JHCPAN

In addition, The President's Marathon Challenge at Tufts coordinates and trains runners for the Boston Marathon as part of a large effort to raise awareness and funds for research and outreach on nutrition and physical activity. If you have any interest in joining our team, go to: tuftsmarathonchallenge.com.

The Tufts University Health & Nutrition Letter, an 8-page monthly newsletter, has been called "the best available source of news and views on nutrition" by *U.S. News & World Report* and has also received accolades from *The New York Times, The Boston Globe,* and the *Columbia Journalism Review,* among other publications. Visit www.healthletter.tufts.edu, or call 800-271-7584.

Books on Back Health and Related Topics

All You Need to Know About Back Pain: Beat Pain, Increase Mobility and Know Your Options. Mary Anne Dunkin (Atlanta: Arthritis Foundation, 2002).

Mind Over Back Pain: A Radically New Approach to the Diagnosis and Treatment of Back Pain. John E. Sarno (New York: Berkley Publishing Group, 1999).

Our Bodies, Ourselves: A New Edition for a New Era. Boston Women's Health Book Collective (New York: Touchstone, 2005).

General Back Health Resources

The American Academy of Physical Medicine and Rehabilitation
    One IBM Plaza, Ste. 2500
    Chicago, IL 60611-3604
    Phone: 312-464-9700
    www.aapmr.org

The American Academy of Physical Medicine and Rehabilitation is the national medical society of physiatrists (doctors who specialize in physical medicine and rehabilitation). The Academy provides information about the care and treatment of back, neck, and spinal cord pain and guidance for locating a physiatrist in your area.

The American Association of Neurological Surgeons
  5550 Meadowbrook Dr.
  Rolling Meadows, IL 60008
  Phone: 847-378-0500
  E-mail: info@aans.org
  www.aans.org
  www.neurosurgerytoday.org

The American Association of Neurological Surgeons (AANS) is an association of board certified neurosurgeons dedicated to advancing neurological surgery. AANS has a helpful Web site with a library of information, the latest research, and a link to locate a board certified neurosurgeon in your area.

Scoliosis Research Society
  555 E. Wells St., Ste. 1100
  Milwaukee, WI 53202-3823
  Phone: 414-289-9107
  E-mail: info@srs.org
  www.srs.org/patients

The Scoliosis Research Society (SRS) is an international society of leading specialists in the research and treatment of spinal deformities. Its Web site provides educational materials for patients both as brochures and online; click on "Patient/Public Information" on the sidebar for resources on scoliosis and how to locate an SRS physician in your area.

General Health Information

Centers for Disease Control and Prevention
  1600 Clifton Rd.
  Atlanta, GA 30333
  Phone: 800-311-3435 TYY: 404-639-3312
  www.cdc.org

The Centers for Disease Control and Prevention (CDC) provides consumers with comprehensive information about nutrition, physical activity, and numerous other health-related topics. The main home page can be a good place to start your search, but I also provide here two more specific areas about exercise and ergonomics.

The CDC on exercise:
National Center for Chronic Disease Prevention and Health Promotion (NCCDPHP); Division of Nutrition and Physical Activity (DNPA)
  4770 Buford Hwy. NE
  Atlanta, GA 30341-3717
  www.cdc.gov/nccdphp/dnpa

The CDC on occupational health:
  The National Institute for Occupational Safety and Health (NIOSH) is part of the Centers for Disease Control and Prevention (CDC). This agency is responsible for conducting research and making recommendations for the prevention of work-related injury and illness, as well as providing information, education, and training in the field of occupational safety and health to the public.
  Phone: 800-356-4674
  http://www.cdc.gov/niosh/topics/ergonomics

Fitness Resources

Stretching: 20th Anniversary. Rev. ed. Bob Anderson (Bolinas, CA: Shelter Publications, 2000). This is the gold standard for stretching exercises.

American College of Sports Medicine
   PO Box 1440
   Indianapolis, IN 46206
   www.acsm.org

The American College of Sports Medicine is an organization that conducts research in the field of exercise science and certifies fitness professionals.

American Council on Exercise
   4851 Paramount Dr.
   San Diego, CA 92123
   Phone: 800-825-3636
   www.acefitness.org

The American Council on Exercise (ACE) is a fitness organization that will help locate certified exercise professionals in your area.

America On the Move
   44 School St., Ste. 325
   Boston, MA 02108
   Phone: 800-807-0077
   www.americaonthemove.org

America On the Move, a national initiative through The Partnership to Promote Healthy Eating and Active Living, is dedicated to helping individuals and communities across the nation make positive changes to improve health and quality of life.

Fifty-Plus Lifelong Fitness
  PO Box 20230
  Stanford, CA 94309
  Phone: 650-323-6160
  www.50plus.org

Fifty-Plus Lifelong Fitness is a national organization whose sole mission is the promotion of physical activity for older adults.

National Strength and Conditioning Association
  1955 N. Union Blvd.
  Colorado Springs, CO 80909
  Phone: 719-632-6722 or 800-805-6826
  www.nsca.com

The National Strength and Conditioning Association Web site lists certified personal trainers.

Ergonomic and Occupational Health Resources
The American Occupational Therapy Association, Inc.
  4720 Montgomery La.
  PO Box 31220
  Bethesda, MD 20824-1220
  Phone: 301-652-2682 or 800-377-8555
  www.aota.org

The Canadian Centre for Occupational Health and Safety (CCOHS)
   135 Hunter St. E.
   Hamilton, ON
   Canada L8N 1M5
   Phone: 800-263-8466
   www.ccohs.ca

The Canadian Centre for Occupational Health and Safety offers a wealth of occupational health and safety resources, including a link for "Ergonomics and Human Factors," which provides extensive information, recommendations, and resources.

Cornell Human Factors and Ergonomics Research Group Dept. Design & Environmental Analysis, College of Human Ecology
   Cornell University
   MVR Hall, Forest Home Dr.
   Ithaca, NY 14853-4401
   Phone: 607-255-1957
   http://ergo.human.cornell.edu

The Cornell Human Factors and Ergonomics Research Group provides information and tips about ergonomic aspects of furniture, equipment, and movement in the home, school, and workplace to improve comfort, performance and health.

Complementary Medicine Information

The Relaxation Response. Herbert Benson, M.D. (New York: Harper-Torch, 1976).

Alexander Technique International
  1692 Massachusetts Ave., 3rd floor
  Cambridge, MA 02138
  Phone: 888-668-8996 or 617-497-5151
  Fax: 617-497-2615
  E-mail: ati-usa@ati-net.com
  www.ati-net.com

Alexander Technique International's Web site provides a wealth of articles, links, and a database of ATI certified teachers, and the online *Journal of Alexander Technique International* (click on "ExchangE"). This is a worldwide organization, with its headquarters located in the USA.

American Society for the Alexander Technique
  PO Box 60008
  Florence, MA 01062
  Phone: 800-473-0620 or 413-584-2359
  E-mail: info@amsat.ws
  www.alexandertech.org

American Society for the Alexander Technique (AmSAT) is the largest professional organization of teachers of the Alexander Technique and maintains a high standard of certification.

American Academy of Medical Acupuncture
    4929 Wilshire Blvd., Ste. 428
    Los Angeles, CA 90010
    Phone: 323-937-5514
    www.medicalacupuncture.org

American Chiropractic Association
    1701 Clarendon Blvd.
    Arlington, VA 22209
    Phone: 800-986-4636
    E-mail: memberinfo@amerchiro.org
    www.amerchiro.org

The American Chiropractic Association is the largest professional association for Doctors of Chiropractic. The main page highlights relevant news stories; click on "Patient Information" and "Publications" for additional information and research updates. There is also a "Find a Doctor of Chiropractic" link at the top of the screen.

American Massage Therapy Association (AMTA)
    500 Davis St., Ste. 900
    Evanston, IL 60201-4695
    Phone: 877-905-2700 or 847-864-0123
    E-mail: info@amtamassage.org
    www.amtamassage.org

American Occupational Therapy Association
    4720 Montgomery La.
    PO Box 31220
    Bethesda, MD 20824-1220
    Phone: 301-652-2682
    www.aota.org

The American Occupational Therapy Association is the nationally recognized professional association of occupational therapists, occupational therapy assistants, and students of occupational therapy. Practitioners work with people experiencing health problems such as spinal cord injuries. The Web site has practical information for consumers.

American Physical Therapy Association
    1111 N. Fairfax St.
    Alexandria, VA 22314-1488
    Phone: 800-999-APTA (2782) or 703-683-6748
    www.apta.org

The American Physical Therapy Association is a national professional organization that promotes the advancement of research, education, and treatment practices. The Web site provides a link to "Information for Consumers," which gives background resources on physical therapy, insurance coverage, news stories, and a link to "Find a PT." The APTA also publishes the *Journal of the American Physical Therapy Association;* the journal can be accessed at www.ptjournal.org.

Commission on Massage Therapy Accreditation
   1007 Church St., Ste. 302
   Evanston, IL 60201
   Phone: 847-869-5039
   E-mail: info@comta.org
   www.comta.org

The Commission on Massage Therapy Accreditation is recognized by the U.S. Department of Education to ensure standards of education, training, and practice for massage therapy. You can browse the Accredited Programs Directory to find out which massage schools are accredited by COMTA in your area.

Feldenkrais Educational Foundation of North America (FEFNA)
   3611 SW Hood Ave., Ste. 100
   Portland, OR 97239
   Phone: 866-333-6248 or 503-221-6612
   www.feldenkrais.com

The Feldenkrais Educational Foundation of North America Web site is operated by the North American Guild of Feldenkrais. Click on "Learn About the Method" for background information, articles, and resources on the Feldenkrais Method. The "Practitioners and Classes" link will allow you to locate a North American Guild of Feldenkrais certified practitioner in your area.

National Certification Commission for Acupuncture and Oriental
Medicine
   11 Canal Center Plaza, Ste. 300
   Alexandria, VA 22314
   Phone: 703-548-9004
   E-mail: info@nccaom.org
   www.nccaom.org

The Pilates Method Alliance
   PO Box 370906
   Miami, FL 33137-0906
   Phone: 866-573-4945
   E-mail: info@pilatesmethodalliance.org
   www.pilatesmethodalliance.org

The Pilates Method Alliance is an international organization for education and certification of Pilates Method professionals.

The Rolf Institute of Structural Integration
   5055 Chaparral Ct., Ste. 103
   Boulder, CO 80301
   Phone: 303-449-5903 or 800-530-8875
   E-mail: info@rolf.org
   www.rolf.org

The Rolfing Institute of Structural Integration is the only certifying
body for Rolf practitioners. The Web site includes background information about the practice of Rolfing and training programs, a link to
locate a certified Rolfer in your area, and recent media articles. Of
particular interest is the section "About Rolfing," where you will see
the topics "Theory and Principles" and "Back Pain."

Tai Chi Productions
  PO Box 752
  Butler, NJ 07405
  Phone: 973-282-9698
  www.taichiproductions.com

Yoga Journal
  Yoga Teachers Directory and Source
  2054 University Ave.
  Berkeley, CA 94704
  Phone: 510-841-9200
  www.yogajournal.com

Exercise Equipment

  Australian Barbell Company
  52-54 Bond St. W.
  Mordialloc, Victoria 3195
  Australia
  E-mail: info@australianbarbellco.com
  www.australianbarbellco.com
  (Click on the "Steps, Mats, Medicine & Fitness Balls" link to pur-
  chase yoga mats and fitness balls.)

Danskin
  530 Seventh Ave.
  New York, NY 10018
  Phone: 800-288-6749
  E-mail: Contact_us@danskin.com
  www.danskin.com
  (Click on "Equipment" and then "Yoga" to purchase yoga mats.)

Gaiam
    360 Interlocken Blvd., Ste 300
    Broomfield, CO 80021
    Phone: 877-989-6321
    E-mail: customerservice@gaiam.com
    www.gaiam.com
    (Under "Mind-Body Fitness" you can purchase a variety of yoga
    mats, resistance-band kits with three levels of resistance, and fit-
    ness balls.)

Strong Women
Get Involved!

◈

There are a number of different ways that women can participate in Strong Women activities. Following is a summary. Whether you're a newcomer to the world of fitness and better health or a longtime Strong Women aficionado, the activities and resources listed here are open to you. We encourage you to explore what's out there, and get and stay involved, for the sake of your physical and emotional health—and also because participating is great fun.

THE STRONGWOMEN™ PROGRAM

The Program's Mission
StrongWomen™ catalyzes positive change in women of all ages to live stronger, healthier lives by providing knowledge, inspiration, access to programs, and ongoing support.

The Program's Vision

StrongWomen™ envisions a worldwide community of members who are fit, strong, and healthy; in turn, these empowered women will become positive agents of change for their families, communities, and beyond.

The Program

Lead by renowned fitness and nutrition researcher and international bestselling author, Miriam Nelson, Ph.D., Tufts University's StrongWomen™ Program is a low-cost, community-based, strength-training program that translates scientific research into practical results. Now,

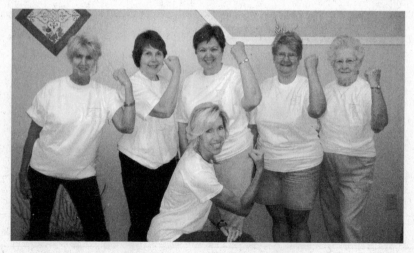

Program participants in Indiana

through an evidence-based curriculum, this program is available in not-for-profit settings around North America. Trained program leaders are emerging across the United States and Canada. Women of all ages, led by these trained leaders in their own communities, are increasingly adopting healthful strategies and reporting dramatic improvements in age-associated conditions such as osteoporosis, arthritis, weight gain, weakness, frailty, and depression.

In response to overwhelming public demand created by her Strong-Women books, Dr. Nelson and colleague Rebecca Seguin, M.S., C.S.C.S., began conducting StrongWomen™ Program workshops to train individuals as program leaders in their own communities throughout the country. With the support of Nelson and Seguin's StrongWomen™ Tool Kit curriculum, these program leaders then spread the StrongWomen™ message that diet and exercise can allow women to remain strong, healthy, and vibrant at any age. Currently, more than 200 StrongWomen™ programs are being offered to several thousand participants throughout thirty-four states as well as Canada.

The StrongWomen™ Program provides a safe, low-cost, and enjoyable social atmosphere where midlife and older women—who might not otherwise take these important steps—can nurture their physical and emotional selves.

Program Benefits

The benefits of strength training for older women have been studied extensively and include:

- Increased muscle mass and strength
- Improved bone density and reduced risk for osteoporosis and related fractures

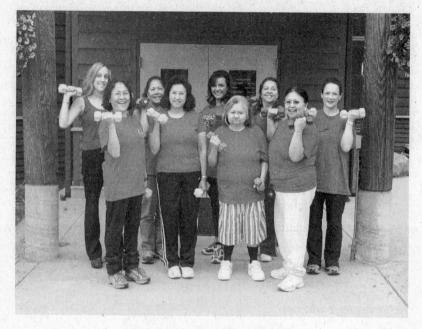

Program participants in Alaska

- Improved control of diabetes, heart disease, arthritis, depression, and body weight
- Improved self-confidence, sleep, and vitality

Where to Find a StrongWomen™ Program Near You

To identify if a StrongWomen™ Program is offered near you, visit: **go.tufts.edu/strongwomen**

STRONGWOMEN™ SUMMITS

Come Share the Experience

Held each year, the popular StrongWomen™ Summits bring together women committed to getting involved—women who want to make a difference in their lives, work, and communities. Dr. Miriam Nelson hosts these inspirational retreats in several venues around the country. The hundreds of women who attend each weekend-long summit come away from these events feeling challenged, engaged, and motivated to adopt a more energized, stronger lifestyle.

Summit attendees learn specific steps to take toward finding joy in their lives; learn humorous insights and stress-management techniques; take part in yoga sessions; and enjoy a little private time as well. With a delicious and healthful menu, this is a weekend-long program to savor and remember. Participants include mothers and daughters, friends and coworkers, as well as those who come solo and make new friends over the course of the weekend. Also offered are practical advice, inspiration, and the empowering knowledge that strength, joy, and vibrant health are within reach at any age.

STRONGWOMEN™ MOUNTAIN SUMMITS

Awesome, Exhilarating, Rejuvenating

Women looking for a life-changing, enabling experience that encourages strength and builds confidence will want to consider these exciting mountain trips. For the last few years, Dr. Nelson has teamed up with internationally recognized guide Isabelle Santoire to lead a select group of women into the mountains and on to a better place—physically, mentally, and spiritually. Participants are able to set their own pace with the warmth, support, and friendship of other Strong-Women™. Rita Henley Jensen, founder and editor in chief of Women eNews and a 2005 StrongWomen™ Mountain Summit participant, says, "Be ready to do what you never dreamed you were capable of—and meet fantastic other women who are willing to do the same.

The climbs are beautifully prepared and exquisitely selected, and the guides are the kindest and most capable. Make friends for life and enjoy the beauty the world offers while learning and improving your health."

StrongWomen™ Mountain Summits are one of the few outdoor adventure programs for women that are developed and led by internationally recognized health experts. They provide women the rare opportunity to benefit from the day-to-day advice, support, and company of leaders who hike, eat, sleep, laugh, and learn with them during the course of a week or more in some of the world's most beautiful settings. The StrongWomen™ Mountain Summits are ideal for women who need a break to reconnect with themselves—body, mind, and spirit—and nature.

For more information visit www.StrongWomen.com.

StrongWomen Web site (www.StrongWomen.com)

For up-to-the-minute information on health, fitness, and emotional well-being, visit Dr. Nelson's Web site. Topics and features include:

- Diet/Nutrition
- Getting Fit
- Workout Tips and Exercises
- Staying Young
- Staying Slim
- Strong Bones
- Chronic Diseases and Other Health Concerns
- Upcoming Events and Talks

StrongWomen e-Newsletter

Also on the StrongWomen Web site, you'll find Dr. Nelson's informative monthly newsletter. Regular features include:

- The latest news in women's health and fitness research
- StrongWomen™'s Summit news
- Mountain Summit trip news
- Public talks and events
- Reader questions and answers on exercise, eating, and more
- Success stories from inspiring women
- Healthful and delicious recipes to try at home

Sign up for the newsletter and get more information on all of the above programs and resources, at www.StrongWomen.com.

LLuminari

Dr. Nelson is a health expert and cofounder of LLuminari. LLuminari manages all of the StrongWomen™ Summits, the Web site StrongWomen.com, and the monthly e-newsletter. LLuminari is a health and wellness company made up of the country's leading health and wellness doctors, scientists, and professionals. They bring the best and brightest together across disciplines—body, mind, and spirit. Evidence-based, charismatic, and creative, LLuminari health experts communicate in ways that change women's lives. Please visit their Web site, www.LLuminari.com, for more information.

Other Books in the Strong Women Series

◆

Despite overwhelming scientific support and recommendations from the U.S. Surgeon General and the American College of Sports Medicine, fewer than 25 percent of women in the United States get the exercise they need. Dr. Miriam Nelson's Strong Women book series was created to address these issues and to spread the message that physical decline is not an inevitable part of aging.

For nearly a decade, Dr. Nelson has been writing accessible, practical health guides tailored for women in midlife and beyond. Published in thirteen languages, her Strong Women books have sold more than a million copies worldwide.

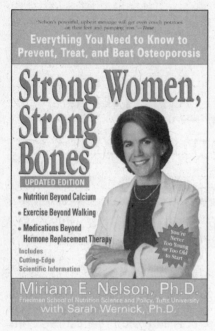

Strong Women, Strong Bones:
Everything You Need to Know
to Prevent, Treat, and
Beat Osteoporosis
Updated edition
By Miriam E. Nelson, Ph.D.,
with Sarah Wernick, Ph.D.

Updated in 2006, this groundbreaking guide to understanding and combating osteoporosis has sold more than 100,000 copies. The book provides detailed, up-to-date information on nutrition, exercise, and medications, including recent FDA findings. Also included is a new two-minute exercise that yields astonishing results.

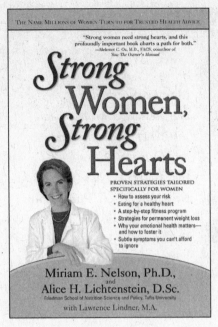

Strong Women, Strong Hearts:
Proven Strategies Tailored
Specifically for Women
By Miriam E. Nelson, Ph.D.,
and Alice H. Lichtenstein, D.Sc.,
with Lawrence Lindner, M.A.

In this practical guide, Dr. Nelson teams up with renowned heart expert Dr. Alice Lichtenstein to present the latest information every woman needs in order to fight heart disease. This is the leading killer of women in the United States and kills *more women than men* each year. Topics include assessing your risk, eating right, a step-by-step fitness program, and hidden factors such as emotional health and hard-to-recognize symptoms unique to women.

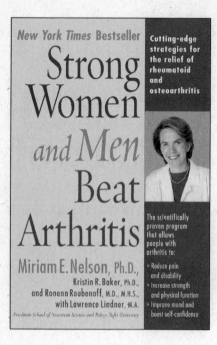

Strong Women and Men *Beat Arthritis: Cutting-Edge Strategies for the Relief of Rheumatoid and Osteoarthritis* By Miriam E. Nelson, Ph.D., Kristin R. Baker, Ph.D., and Ronenn Roubenoff, M.D., M.H.S., with Lawrence Lindner, M.A.

A *New York Times*–bestselling guide for anyone who suffers from arthritis, this book provides a simple strength-training program that has been proven to reduce pain and inflammation. Also included is a scientifically based eating plan, a guide to the latest medications, and the real story on complementary therapies, revealing which ones truly work.

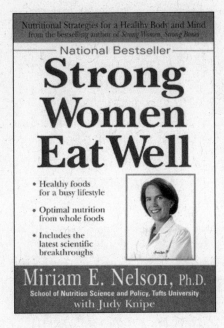

Strong Women Eat Well:
Nutritional Strategies for a
Healthy Body and Mind
By Miriam E. Nelson, Ph.D.,
with Judy Knipe

A national bestseller that sets the record straight on eating for good health, including everything you need to know to read nutrition labels, choose the right eating plan to fit your needs, and take the right dietary supplements. Included are fifty delicious, easy-to-prepare recipes.

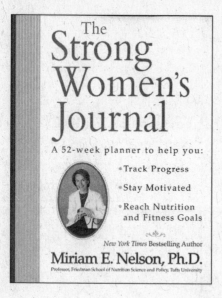

The Strong Women's Journal
By Miriam E. Nelson, Ph.D.

How many reps? How much calcium? How many calories? How many miles? A perfect companion to the bestselling Strong Women books, this 52-week journal helps readers keep track of progress, goals, and daily exercise and eating patterns, as well as individual thoughts and feelings along the way. More than a journal, the book includes essential advice and information to help the reader achieve lasting results.

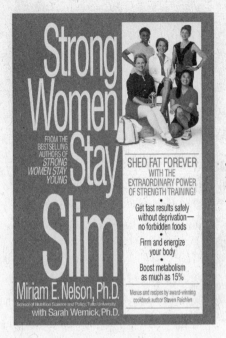

Strong Women Stay Slim
By Miriam E. Nelson, Ph.D.,
with Sarah Wernick, Ph.D.

This popular guide presents a proven program for boosting metabolism and shedding pounds, for all ages and fitness levels. With fully illustrated exercises designed specifically for weight loss, along with a hunger-free food plan that includes menus and recipes, the book helps readers get and stay on track for better health and a slimmer figure.

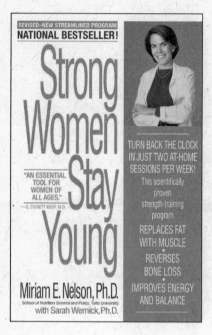

Strong Women Stay Young
Revised edition
By Miriam E. Nelson, Ph.D.,
with Sarah Wernick, Ph.D.

A bestseller in its first edition, this groundbreaking guide presents a scientifically proven strength-training program for women thirty-five and up. The revised edition features eight streamlined exercises with fully illustrated instructions; new supplemental moves for the back, abs, and more; a complete program to do at the gym, and an all-new chapter for men. Significant improvements can be seen after just four weeks.

Strong Women health guides are available wherever books are sold. To obtain more information, visit www.StrongWomen.com or www.penguin.com.

Acknowledgments

◈

For all their help in so many ways, I want to thank my colleagues at Tufts University. I could not have written this book without the support, in particular, of those at the Friedman School of Nutrition Science and Policy and all the faculty, staff, and students affiliated with the John Hancock Center for Physical Activity and Nutrition.

To the funders of our work at Tufts, especially John Hancock Financial Services, Inc., and the New Balance Foundation, I also express deep gratitude.

My appreciation goes as well to my colleagues at Putnam for putting themselves behind this project. Marian Lizzi, my very talented editor, championed this book from start to finish. Wendy Wray, my patient illustrator, continues to provide graceful and instructive artwork for my books. For my agent, Wendy Weil, thanks, as always, for everything. You are the best there is!

Others to whom I owe a debt of gratitude for their longtime support include my colleagues at LLuminari, especially Elizabeth Browning, for managing all of my StrongWomen efforts; Gary Hirshberg and his team at Stonyfield Farm; and Neill Walsdorf Jr. of Mission Pharmacal.

Four individuals who directly assisted in the writing of this book include Sandra Klemmer, my incredible editorial assistant, who provided valuable input, review, and feedback throughout the process, and also served as one of the models for the illustrations; Michael Pimentel, CSCS, LATC, director of Strength/Conditioning & Fitness at Tufts University, who was instrumental in helping me develop the book's exercise program; Barry Pailet, MS, LMT, massage therapist, who assisted me with the chapter on complementary medicine; and Rina Bloch, M.D., physical medicine and rehabilitation specialist at Tufts–New England Medical Center, who vetted the manuscript and provided invaluable commentary and suggestions. (Any errors that might be found in this book are mine, not hers.)

For their own "back" stories, much thanks go to Amanda, Anne, Christina, Josephine, Molly, and Rhonda. In addition, thank you to Amelia Winslow and Francis Otting, who served as models for the illustrations.

Finally, both my writing collaborator, Larry Lindner, and I would like to thank our patient families for their support throughout the writing process; in particular, our spouses, Kin Earle and Constance Lindner, and our children, Mason, Eliza, Alexandra, and John Matthew. You all are the backbone that keeps us well aligned.

Index

ABOUT THE AUTHORS

Miriam Nelson, Ph.D., is Director of the John Hancock Center for Physical Activity and Nutrition and Associate Professor of Nutrition at the Friedman School of Nutrition Science and Policy at Tufts University. She is also a fellow of the American College of Sports Medicine, an honor reserved for those who have demonstrated leadership and research in the field of exercise.

For the last seventeen years, Dr. Nelson has been principal investigator of studies on exercise and nutrition, work supported by grants from the government and private foundations. During this time she was named a Brookdale National Fellow, a prestigious award given annually to only five or six young scholars deemed to be future leaders in the field of aging. She was also awarded a Bunting Fellowship at the Mary Ingraham Bunting Institute at Radcliffe College. In 1998, Dr. Nelson received the Lifetime Achievement Award from the Massachusetts Governor's Committee on Physical Fitness and Sports, and in 2005, she received the Woman of Valor award from the American Diabetes Association. The following year, she was presented with an award from the New England Chapter of the American Medical Writers Association for her work in communicating the importance of nutrition and fitness to women.

Dr. Nelson is the author of the international bestsellers *Strong Women Stay Young; Strong Women Stay Slim; Strong Women, Strong Bones; Strong Women Eat Well; Strong Women* and Men *Beat Arthritis; the Strong Women's Journal;* and *Strong Women, Strong Hearts.*

These titles, published in fourteen languages, have sold more than a million copies worldwide. *Strong Women, Strong Bones* received the esteemed Books for a Better Life Award for best wellness book of 2000 from the Multiple Sclerosis Society.

In August 2001, Dr. Nelson appeared in her own PBS special entitled *Strong Women Live Well*, which focused on the benefits of exercise and nutrition for women's health. She has been featured on many television and radio shows, including *The Oprah Winfrey Show*, *Today*, *Good Morning America*, *ABC Nightly News*, CNN, *Fresh Air*, and the Discovery Channel. A motivational speaker who lectures about women's health around the world, she is also a LLuminari health expert. She lives in Concord, Massachusetts, with her husband and three children.

Lawrence Lindner, M.A., has written several books on health and other topics. He also penned the "Eating Right" column for the *Washington Post* for several years and currently freelances for a variety of magazines and newspapers. He lives in Hingham, Massachusetts, with his wife and son.

To contact Dr. Nelson, please send letters to:
Miriam E. Nelson, Ph.D.
Director, John Hancock Center for Physical Activity and Nutrition
Friedman School of Nutrition Science and Policy
Tufts University
150 Harrison Ave.
Boston, MA 02111
Dr. Nelson regrets that due to the volume of mail she receives, she cannot respond personally to every letter.

Please visit: www.strongwomen.com

DATE			
1/29/85			

RED SHADOWS

The aim of Zenith Books is to present the history of minority groups in the United States and their participation in the growth and development of the country. Through histories and biographies written by leading historians in collaboration with established writers for young people, Zenith Books will increase awareness of and at the same time develop an understanding and appreciation for minority group heritage.

DR. JOHN HOPE FRANKLIN, Chairman of the History Department at the University of Chicago, has also taught at Brooklyn College, Fisk University, and Howard University. For the year 1962–63, he was William Pitt Professor of American History and Institutions at Cambridge University in England. He is the author of many books, including *From Slavery to Freedom*, *The Militant South*, *Reconstruction After the Civil War*, and *The Emancipation Proclamation*.

DAN GEORGAKAS was born in Detroit, Michigan. He attended Wayne State University, where he received a B.A. degree in history, and the University of Michigan, where he received his M.A. degree. In 1963, Mr. Georgakas was a member of a Fulbright Study group in Greece. His poetry has appeared in the following anthologies: *Where Is Vietnam*, *31 New American Poets*, *The Now Generation*, *Campfires of the Resistance*, *Thunderbolts of Peace and Freedom*, and many more. Currently, Mr. Georgakas is working on a book on the recent history of the city of Detroit and also a novel.

Another outstanding Zenith Book

The Broken Hoop, by Dan Georgakas. The history of native Americans from 1600 to 1890, from the Atlantic Coast to the Plains.

RED SHADOWS

The history of Native Americans
from 1600 to 1900, from
the desert to the Pacific Coast

DAN GEORGAKAS

ZENITH BOOKS
DOUBLEDAY & COMPANY, INC., GARDEN CITY, NEW YORK

The Zenith Books edition, published simultaneously in hard-bound and paperback volumes, is the first publication of *Red Shadows*.

Zenith Books Edition: 1973
ISBN: 0-385-06889-1 Trade
       0-385-06916-2 Paperbound
Library of Congress Catalog Card Number 74–175375
9 8 7 6 5 4 3

COVER CREDIT: Navajo blanket with twelve figures from Navajo, New Mexico, courtesy of Museum of the American Indian, Heye Foundation, New York, New York.

1977

970.1
GEO

CONTENTS

INTRODUCTION

When Columbus discovered America in 1492, he called it the New World. Five hundred years before Columbus, roving Vikings had discovered America and called it Vineland. Thousands of years before the Vikings, Phoenicians and possibly Egyptians may have discovered America when blown off course by storms. But at least ten thousand years before any of these explorers, the ancestors of the Indians had been the first people to discover America. They became the Native Americans.

Most scholars believe the Native Americans' ancestors crossed from Siberia to Alaska by means of what was then either a land bridge or short waterway between Asia and North America. One skull found in California indicates that these people may have been living in North America as early as 20,000 B.C. At another place what appears to be a man-made fireplace dates back to 30,000 B.C.

By the time of Columbus, the Native Americans had developed over two thousand languages and major dialects, more than in all of Europe and Asia. Rather than alphabets, Indians used picture symbols to help their remarkable memories retain their rich oral tradition of songs, stories, poetry, and rituals. Their eloquence has become renowned. Wherever possible in the pages that follow, direct quotes and Indian poetic imagery will be utilized. The earth will be Great Painted Lady. Citizens of the

United States will be people of the eagle. Concepts such as *forever* will be put in the Indian form as *long as the grass shall grow and the water flow.*

The Native Americans greeted the first Europeans with friendship and hospitality. Their legends told of a tribe of lost white brothers who would some day be reunited with them. The Indians were hurt and then angered when the white people did not act as brothers. The white tribes wanted to destroy Indian religion and to make Indians work as slaves. They wanted to take away minerals and to possess land. The Native Americans believed there was great harmony in the universe, but they could not understand how the white people fit into that harmony. The advance of the Europeans seemed to destroy the order of the ages. First the eastern woodlands, the swamps, and the plains, then the desert, the coast, and the mountains of the West were overrun and parceled out by the whites. The buffalo were slaughtered and the salmon depleted. Disease and war killed off the majority of Indians. The others were forced on reservations where their traditions were systematically destroyed. The last survivor of one of the California tribes put it simply, "You stay, I go." But as Chief Seattle of the Spokane prophesied, the spirits of the departed linger. By the banks of lonely rivers and in the wilderness of steel canyons, red shadows whisper there are other ways of living than we now live and other ways of dreaming than we now dream.

Banks of the Musconetcong
Delaware Country
1973

Part I

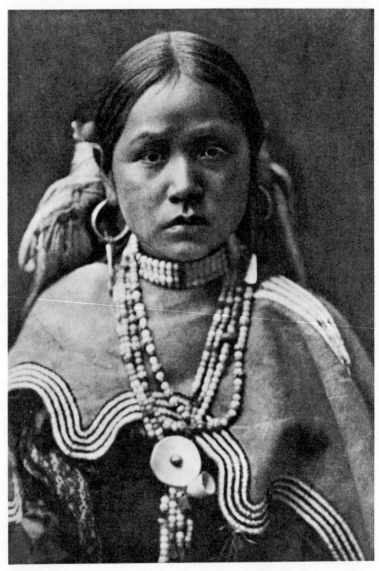

Young Apache girl wearing her finest traditional clothing and jewelry. (*Huntington Free Library, Heye Foundation*)

Great Painted Lady:
THE SOUTHWEST

*If the Great Father wants my braves
to cease attacks across the Texas
border, he will have to remove
Texas far enough away so my young
men cannot find it.*

Satanta (Kiowa)

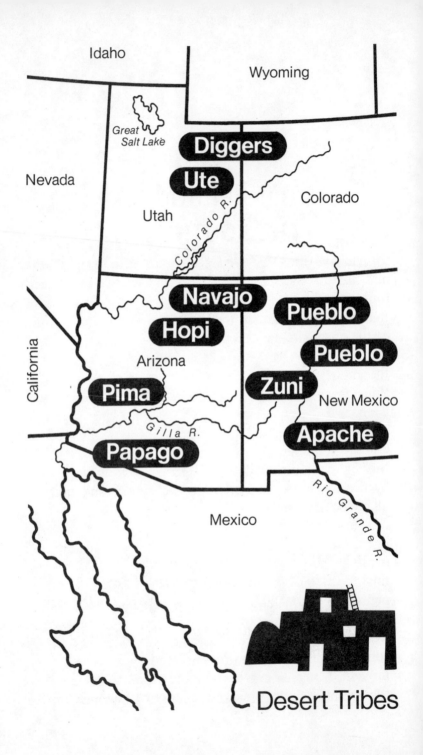

Desert Tribes

LAND OF THE SUN

Vast plateaus seem to roll forever under the all powerful sun. In the distance, mountains peak to elegant heights and almost touch the clear blue that carries magnificent thunderhead clouds that only too rarely release the rains that never quite satisfy the endless thirst of the parched earth. The white dunes sometimes take a blood red color or become painted deserts. It is a vast and quiet region, but to the Indians who made it their home, there was no such thing as emptiness. Everything was alive with spirit power. Even the heavens above were filled with the wandering souls of the dead and numberless supernatural beings. Only in some remote spot or in some sheltered silence of the night could the voices of these spirits be heard. Only by tireless contemplation could the totality and unity of all life be understood.

Where mountains intruded into the heat, the Indians knew they might find forests of aspen and the rich soil made by ancient lava flows. Caves inside such mountains might contain bats and ice, yet outside the sun was supreme. Occasionally lightning storms might crack the sky with white stitches of thunder and lightning, but the southwest desert, the area that became New Mexico and Arizona, primarily meant endless miles of wind-eroded, thirsting soil. Canyons cut by creeping rivers that were older than mankind made sudden plunges thousands of feet deep, the canyon walls a geological record of the time between the present and the ages before the dinosaurs. It was here the Grand Canyon had been carved, and it was here the colors were so spectacular the Indians called the earth Great Painted Lady.

Unlike the Indians of the eastern woodlands who created large political units such as the Iroquois League of the Five Nations, the people of the Southwest tended to live in small groups. In the southern part of Arizona around the Gila River there were cities of the Pima or River People. Directly to the south of them in the deserts were the Papago or Desert People. In New Mexico, the most important tribes were the Pueblo, who took their name from the style of homes they built. Some of the most famous of their cities were Zuñi, Taos, and the seven villages of the Hopi. To the east of the Pueblo where the deserts begin to give way to prairies, there were raiding tribes such as the Kiowa and Comanche who lived in the manner of the Plains people. To the west along the Colorado River, which is now one of the borders of California, there were the fierce Yuma and Mohave. But in New Mexico and Arizona, people were not much interested in war. The Hopi's name for themselves was Hopitu, the peaceful people. Warriors rarely bothered to hunt the scarce game of the arid region and the few weapons were mainly used for self-defense and occasional fights to show individual bravery.

The Southwesterners were essentially farming people. They had developed their agriculture to such a degree that they never had to worry about having enough food and thus had much leisure time for the dancing and singing they loved so much. Sometime around the year A.D. 1000 new tribes called Apache and Navajo entered the area. These newcomers from the North possessed a more advanced type of bow, and they wore skins and leather moccasins. They were much less organized than the farmers and rarely had permanent homes. They lived in deep canyons with good hiding places from which to base attacks on their prosperous neighbors. The raiders were often identified by their secondary or subtribal names, which usually came from the area they lived in. Among such names for the Apache were Mescalero Apache, Chiricahua Apache, and White Mountain Apache. A group of Apache even became officially adopted by the Kiowa and became known as Kiowa Apache. The raiders were not united by any government but felt a certain relationship because of similar languages and customs.

THE RAIN LOVERS

By the time Columbus touched America, the Pima and the Papago had been living in the same places for over three thousand years. They had built complicated irrigation canals to store water for their crops. Hunting and war were minimized, and men devoted their main energies to agriculture. Special varieties of maize or corn were developed with ceremonial significance attached to each type. These decentralized farmers were peaceful people. Survival was so dependent upon the rain that every ceremony and ritual, even those having to do with war, was tied to the need for rain. The Pima and Papago did not enjoy being warriors. Rather than speaking of personal bravery, a Papago warrior chanted how he had seized the enemy's "seeds and beautiful clouds and beautiful winds." All this disagreeable violence was for the purpose of guaranteeing the corn crop.

An important war song ends not with glorification of the
killer but with a hymn to corn:

> *Then came forth a thick stalk and a thick tassel*
> *and the undying seed ripened.*
> *This I did to serve the people.*
> *This should you also think and desire,*
> *all you who are my kinsmen.*

   The supernatural world of the Pima was ruled by Elder
Brother, who had created people out of clay. Ceremonies
often consisted of the retelling and acting out of his splen-
did deeds. The Pima also were in awe of animal spirits,
which could communicate with both men and women, giving them special powers. The animal spirits had the important task of giving dreams. The rain lovers developed
many rituals for these spirits and for Elder Brother. They
often made an offering of prayer sticks. Among some
groups the prayer sticks were made of eagle-feather down,
which represented rain-bringing clouds. These prayer sticks
were often decorated with sacred charms and symbols of
wealth to indicate the giver's appreciation of the gift of
rain. The sticks were sometimes left upon ceremonial
grounds or important springs to indicate in what place the
rain was desired. During rituals, basket drums were played
in the belief that they were calling the clouds to council.
One of the Pima songs which accompanied this music has
the following passage:

> *hi-ya naiho-o! Pluck out the soft down*
> *from the breast of the eagle and turn it*
> *toward the west where small clouds sail*
> *hi-ya naiho-o! beneath the home*
> *of the rain gods it is thundering;*
> *large corn is there. hi-ya naiho-o!*

beneath the home of the rain gods
it is raining; small corn is there.

One of the most fertile areas of the corn growers was the irrigated Gila Valley of Arizona, where the crop was insured by an intricate and rational use of water. The villagers of the Gila had a drinking festival in which they filled themselves with a beerlike alcohol just as the land was supposed to fill itself with water. Their shamans or medicine men had authority only because of dream power and because they were thought to be born with crystals within their bodies that helped them heal. Women were sometimes thought to have crystals but were usually restricted to healing children or helping at the time of birth. Shamans might lose their crystals or have them taken away if they did something incorrectly. Shamans knew good songs to help in a cure, and there were special healing singers for diseases caused by animals. Often disease was thought to come from doing a ritual incorrectly or having broken a taboo. These psychological treatments were accompanied by an impressive knowledge of curative herbs and potions. Ultimately, the Pima and Papago were very practical about medicine. If a shaman had a poor history of curing, he was suspected of being an evil magician or a fake and could be clubbed to death.

The clouds brought rain and the rain brought up the corn. People dreamed of the wonderful spirits in the skies, of all the marvels of their Great Painted Lady. Their poetry expressed complex emotions through simple sentences and sounds. Each word was designed to set off a chain reaction of connected thoughts in the listening imagination. Contrasts and repetitions allowed the individual to reflect on the many subtleties involved in a single word. Songs were creative acts between humans and not entertainment by a few for many. The curing song was part of the cure, just as the rain song was part of the actual cause of rain. Nothing disturbed them so much as to discover that the corn grew just as well for the songless whites. Nor could they understand how whites admired Indian songs without believing in their spiritual content. Creative expression and life were a unity. No other way was safe for the soul or the flesh.

The first known white people to intrude upon the rain lovers were the Spanish. Coronado touched Pima villages in 1540 during his futile search for the legendary Seven Cities of Gold. The decisive personality, however, was Father Kino, a Jesuit missionary who made evangelical tours in 1687. He baptized Pima by the hundreds and gave them Christian names. His work was made easier by the legends which told of a lost tribe of white brothers who were destined to return and help their Indian relatives. The black robe certainly had good magic. He had water rituals, magical names, a new crop called wheat, and fine new cattle. The Papago on the desert heard about the crusader and were eager to find out more about the teachings of the black robes. They began to make a yearly holiday out of going to Mexico to refresh their Christian water names and get beads and other magic charms. A hundred years passed without much change in Indian life. Mexico won independence from Spain in 1823, but the Pima and Papago barely noticed. Not even the coming of settlers from the United States created any difficulty. The newcomers were few in number and were uninterested in the places where the Indians lived. Only the defeat of Mexico by the United States in 1848 caused the first ripples of change. Now, the Pima and most of the Papago were under the direct rule of the United States. A few Pima became scouts for the United States during the war and continued afterwards in new wars against Indians, especially the Apache.

The pony soldiers liked the Pima but were annoyed at the long purification rites required when a warrior happened to kill a foe.

The Pima never made war on the United States and they were proud to boast they did not know the color of a white man's blood. Their territory continued to be outside the major arenas of white interest and ambition. They were farmers who did not object to quiet reservation life in the way the fierce Navajo and Apache did. There would have been little difficulty in bringing such peaceful, productive, and co-operative folk into an interdependent but equal relationship with the white system. But the greed of the whites would not permit it. Everything must be done as they wanted it done. Land must belong to individuals, not groups. Land must be bought and sold like a basket. Since the Pima did not resist, it was a simple matter to draw water from their rivers until the Indian canals went dry. No abrupt or startling event marked the end of Pima prosperity, but as the year 1900 approached, the Pima farms had to be abandoned. The Pima learned English. They adopted the white man's clothing, the white man's housing, and the white man's religion, yet the whites continued to regard them as inferiors. The once proud and wealthy Pima were reduced to poverty.

The Papago fared no better. After the Spanish came, they added wheat crops to their fields of corn. They bred herds of horses and cattle. They fought against the Apache. These changes in the old ways were minimal, but the coming to power of the United States was another matter. That meant reservations, and reservations meant moving to poor land and becoming impoverished. Rather than being prosperous farmers of their own lands, the Papago had to work in cotton fields for daily wages. Traditional clan relationships broke down into desperate individual struggles to survive. Physical comforts built up over centuries diminished. The unity and sympathy of tribal life became an unraveled cord. Like the Pima they withdrew into apathy as they grew poorer while watching the whites grow richer. Like the Pima, they drank too much. Like the Pima, they withdrew into a world of daydreams and memories. Like the Pima, they became listless. Their suffering was less dramatic but no less intense than that of the regal warrior societies of the plains. The world of the buffalo hunters had ended with a bang, the world of the rain lovers with a sigh.

THE PEACEFUL PEOPLE

The Pueblo lived north of the corn growers and took their name from the cliff dwellings of terraced apartments in which they lived. Villages containing hundreds of dwellings lined great streams or were built high on ragged cliffs like Acoma, the sky city. The Pueblo grew many kinds of crops but most important was corn. Their myth of creation spoke of a Sky Father who spread his hand palm downward over the earth and in every wrinkle of his skin there was a shining grain of yellow corn: "In the dark of the early world-dawn, they gleamed like sparks of fire."

Like their neighbors, the Pueblo were concerned with how to bring rain. Their prayers were not spontaneous expressions of an agitated soul but carefully memorized requests for a good life free of violence and drought. Rather than speak of their own personal affairs, the Pueblo sang of the movements of the sun, the problems of the different seasons, and the need that there be enough rain. Their beautiful songs and pageants did not celebrate the individual but the community. Anyone who thought of personal power was considered evil or insane.

The most beloved supernaturals were called the kachinas, two hundred happy cloud and rain beings. Special kachina societies impersonated these spirits by wearing masked costumes and frequently appearing in the plazas or at special events. The Pueblo felt they had a special relationship to these beings. If they fulfilled all their obligations, the rain would fall. The small kachina dolls now admired by tourists represent the full-scale costumes but have no sacred value. Originally, such dolls were used to teach the young about the special characteristics of individual kachinas.

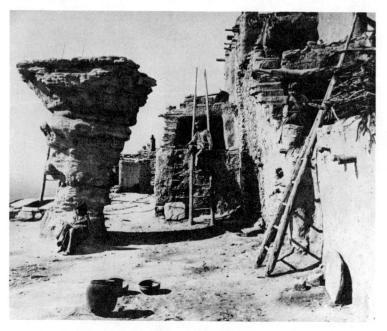

People rest from their chores for a moment on one of the terraces of the Laguna Pueblo in 1879. (*National Archives*)

The Pueblo clowns were almost as popular as the kachinas. These beings who were dressed in amusing costumes were thought to be so mighty that they could say any blasphemy or obscenity they desired. They specialized in custard-pie-in-the-face type humor and jokes about love-making. Very often they were used by the community as a friendly method of criticizing a citizen for vanity or some other shortcoming.

The kachinas, clowns, and other ceremonial figures were controlled by priestly groups organized by strict regulations. Different sets of medicine men controlled different ceremonies and diseases under rights similar to modern patents, licenses, and copyrights. There was little room for the democratic and often egotistical spirit of the plains which sought direct communication with the spirits. The Pueblo man and woman found their worth in a group effort that meshed with what seemed to be a cosmic order. The pageantry of Pueblo ceremonies was a rare art form involving a whole community in laughter, reverence, and happiness. The appearance of the rain gods during one ceremony at the San Juan pueblo has been described thusly:

> Suddenly a deafening noise breaks loose from behind the blanket screen; the closely packed, dimly lit room stirs with joyful anticipation. There is a wild roar from the top of the room where the gods seem to have dropped suddenly, bringing with them frightening thunder, lovely bird songs & cricket chirps & the rhythmic jingling of a hundred tiny bells attached to their writhing waists and swiftly moving feet. The shrill hoots, the resounding whooping & the weird piercing sound which identify each individual rain god intermingle.

Life among the Pueblo was filled with such stirring events. Food was ample and shelter was comfortable, making Pueblo life among the most pleasant in all the Americas. The lack of hunting and war deaths meant males were not maimed or given to short lives. Courtship was minimal and divorce easy. Romance was not much talked about, but it was part of the ordinary life of the married and unmarried, with the same set of rules for women and men. Women had a certain power in that a man came to live in her house when they married. The husband usually kept his ceremonial property and other valuables at his mother's in case of trouble. Should the marriage work out, a man did not become an authoritarian father to his children but a friend and adviser, a role he also took with his sister's children.

Competition and violence were discouraged among the Pueblo. People even wore similar clothing to avoid jealousy. Life was bound to communal needs of the clan. At the time of marriage, clans, not individuals, gave gifts, and in case of marital problems, the clan advised. This vast and close-knit society based on blood ties and marriage vows made the Pueblo individual feel lost and naked when he had to act as a solitary striver in the white man's system of brutal competition.

The Pueblo had little fear of death. They believed the dead ones became clouds and would return with rain. Even so, the Pueblo felt a terrible loss when a loved one died. Members of the family might mourn for four seasons, sitting away from the common fire and rarely finding the energy to speak. The forceful, dominating, and explosive personality valued by the Europeans was unwelcome here. Pueblo society was based on many small cells, each having a mutual respect for all the differing parts. All were equally important and honored just as the ant and the mountain were equally honored in their religion. Hopi sand paintings were started on the outer edges and completed at the center. This gift of encircling and concentrating characterized Pueblo life. Their poetry was religious and their religion was poetic. They did not recite words but sang feelings. Sound was a power in and of itself. The method of the Pueblo was different from that of Europeans but the ultimate goal of happiness was much the same. One ceremony ended with a sacred figure saying,

> *Everything is open*
> *now go home*
> *& leave your worries*
> *& your tears*
> *& sadness.*

And the people responded,

> *Yes, oh yes, yes, yes.*

The mystic Pueblo had a legend of a tribe of lost brothers and they were overjoyed when the Spanish rode into their lives in 1540. This joy soon soured as the Spanish treated them brutally and tried to turn each Pueblo city into a conquered domain. The Pueblo learned about new fruit, vegetables, and tools, but the Spanish would not allow them horses. The Spanish imposed taxes which could be paid in labor time, crops, or finished products such as cloth. Catholicism was forced upon them, and the beloved masked dances forbidden. The Pueblo reasoned these were not the lost white brothers after all but some other tribe. Their gentle nature recoiled at Spanish cruelty, and in the great rebellion of 1680, they rose up and drove all the Spanish from their lands. The victory was short-lived, as the Spanish came back with more soldiers, and in ten years of ruthless combat they re-established their power.

The Spanish were heartless in their manner of ruling,

even cutting off arms and legs to prevent revolt. Many of the Pueblo went to live with the Navajo for safety, but eventually they realized the Spanish were going to remain. Some allowed the newcomers to protect them from raiders such as the Apache, and a few accepted Christianity. The passage of power from Spain to Mexico meant little to the Pueblo, but in 1848 when the United States seized the territory from Mexico, there was a new crisis. Other conquering powers had always recognized Pueblo civilization. The new rulers did not. They considered the Pueblo to be an inferior, stupid, and worthless race.

The Pueblo found themselves forced to take smaller and smaller reservations. The Navajo, their sometime allies, sometime enemies, became more numerous and more powerful until the Pueblo reservations were only pebbles in Navajo ponds. In spite of all hardships and setbacks, the Pueblo's religiously centered government survived. The Pueblo believe they know the secret of the universe. They are convinced a supreme world order of peace such as that long promised to them will be achieved. They resist any attempt to tamper with their ancient beliefs. They do not seek worldly power as most nations do. Power has never been their way. The Pueblo prefer to wait. Like oriental mystics, they feel much can be accomplished by doing nothing. Their patience is not a thing of minutes or days or even the two hundred years of the United States.

THE GREAT LEARNERS

The Apache and Navajo probably came from the northern lake tribes of Canada or Alaska if not from the Asian continent itself. The marauders were ignorant and possessed few material things. They lived by raiding and attempted to learn some of the skills of the Pueblo. The Navajo like most Indian tribes called themselves *the people* (*Dene*) but a more appropriate name for them might be the Great Learners for in a short period of time they would profoundly adapt their way of life twice, first under the influence of other Indians, then under the influence of the whites.

The Pueblo Revolt of 1680 cleared the Southwest of Spaniards as the usually peaceful village folk rose up against their conquerors. The Navajo had little to do with the actual rebellion, but when the Spanish renewed their conquests many of the Pueblo groups sought sanctuary with them. These Pueblo favorably and decisively altered the Navajo way of life. The Pueblo refugees often took Navajo mates, and the Pueblo partner always was the teacher. Agriculture underwent dramatic improvement. Houses changed. The quality of life was refined in a hundred subtle ways with the introduction of sheep flocks marking a basic change from the dependence on raiding. New clans came into existence. Even the Navajo physical type changed as plump figures with small hands and feet like the Pueblo became as common as the tall rangy builds that had previously characterized the tribe. The Navajo took the Pueblo mythology and rituals and added imaginative elements of their own. They were less concerned with rain as they had been hunters and fighters who did not even know the comforts of permanent settlements. They developed special songs and rituals to guarantee the health and luck of their hunters. Previously medicine men had visions which took them to spirit villages where they learned powerful songs and other magic. Now the medicine men adopted elaborate chants for their specific supplications. By 1770 this contact began to break off as the Pueblo returned to their old homes, but the Navajo bands in the nearby canyons were now bursting with new energy and consciousness. Their fighting men were ready for conquests. Their first period of learning was done. Raiding, weaving, agriculture, and trading had made them wealthy and now their herds of sheep and horses would give them a glorious afternoon in the southwest sun.

The Navajo had never had much contact with the Zuñi or Hopi Pueblos and thus felt free to plunder them at will. They raided with an intensity that expressed their determination never to experience poverty again. The most pathetic victims of Navajo warfare were the Diggers, who lived to the north in the area of the Salt Lake Basin. These people were probably the most miserable Indians in North America. They received their name from the fact that they dug roots from the desert floor in order to survive. They were so close to starvation most of the time that they developed almost no poetry, ritual, or social organization. The Diggers could offer no military resistance to the other tribes who took them to sell as slaves. Winter left them so weak and helpless, they actually had to be fattened up in order to survive the trip to places such as Santa Fe where trading for slaves went on. The Diggers were only victims in the slave trade but the Navajo, Apache, Comanche, Ute, Kiowa, and Mexicans were both raiders and raided upon.

Slavery in the West differed greatly from slavery on the plantations of the South. Among the Navajo, female slaves were usually given menial jobs or forced to tend sheep so that Navajo women could do the more intricate task of weaving. Many female slaves became wives, and children who were captured were often adopted as a member of the family. Adult males were not treated nearly so well. Slaves, especially women, were also traded for horses and sheep, which were an important base of wealth. The Navajo fought fiercely to get their share and to defend what they had, but their lives were not centered on war or slavery. One of their night chants has all the calmness of the peaceful Pueblo:

> *In beauty I walk*
> *With beauty before me I walk*
> *With beauty behind me I walk*
> *With beauty above me I walk*
> *With beauty above and about me I walk*
> *It is finished in beauty.*
> *It is finished in beauty.*

The Navajo who were taken as slaves by other Indians were treated pretty much as Navajo treated their own captives. Mexican owners were a bit different. They were more likely to treat female captives as mistresses rather than wives, and they were not very quick to adopt slave children as their own. Male slaves usually became fieldworkers although a lucky few picked up valuable skills which they taught to their own people if they were fortunate enough to escape. The willingness to learn something new, whether it was a skill in working precious metals such as gold or just learning to operate a new machine, was a characteristic of the Navajo. The only thing the Great Learners remained absolutely closed to was the Catholic Church. They simply would not convert.

Few Navajo had had any contact with the United States before 1846 when Kearny's Army of the West entered their lands as part of the Mexican War. These Missouri volunteers were not the usual type of soldier. They elected their own officers, and when Kearny asked them to march in dress uniform, they voted a resolution informing him that they had come to fight, not parade. This army wanted to make allies of the Navajo. The Indians were impressed with them as the soldiers gave good gifts, promised important privileges, and treated them as equals. At one meeting the Navajo and soldiers were even able to feast and dance together. The sounds of tom-toms, clapping hands, rattles, and whistling mingled before the campfire in a strange moment of friendship. Even so, the citizens of the parliamentary republic had no sense of the nature of the democracy they were encountering, a democracy in which no man could ever dictate to any other. Some of the Navajo resented the Americans as late-comers in the long struggle against the Mexicans, but as always, they were willing to acquire valuable allies, especially if they could be protected from other tribes. The Missourians voted to proceed to the interior of Navajo country where they spoke with all the important bands and made a favorable impression. Unfortunately there were too few soldiers to defend the Navajo and the democratic spirit of Kearny's men did not accurately reflect the policies of the United States. Other tribes continued to harass the Navajo. Mexicans continued to raid. The new allies themselves began to issue orders, often contradictory, often shifting from moon to moon. Before long, the Navajo decided to treat the bluecoats as they would any other powerful people. They would fight when cornered, raid when convenient, and flee when outnumbered. The United States soon understood that soldiers would have to be permanently stationed in Navajo country. In a spot the Indians called Green-Place-in-the-Rocks, the bluecoats built a stronghold named Fort Defiance.

The new fort made raiding more difficult but did not alter basic patterns. A few bands made peace, but ten years after the fort was built most Navajo still felt free to attack not only settlers but the fort itself. These bands were delighted when they heard the bluecoats had deserted Fort

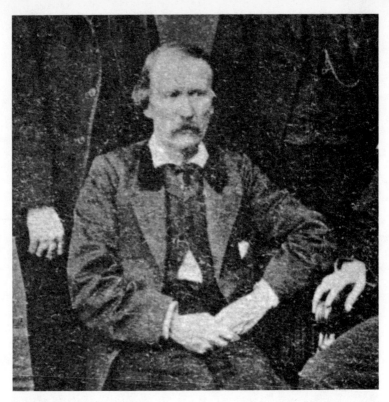

Kit Carson, the army scout, destroyed Navajo herds and placed the people on reservations in 1863. (*Courtesy of Museum of the American Indian, Heye Foundation*)

Defiance. It was the first year of the Civil War and the soldiers were being recalled to fight against other whites, but the Navajo thought their own raids had finally exhausted the pony soldiers and driven them back to the lands they had come from. Emboldened by their "victory," the Navajo raided as never before. Sometimes approached by parties of soldiers in blue and sometimes by soldiers wearing a new gray uniform, the Navajo fought for their own ends in their own ways. They imagined the Southwest was to be their domain forever, but like so many nations at the height of their military might, the confident

Navajo did not know they were enjoying their last summer of power.

The Navajo upsurge was so devastating, the whites decided they must be dealt with at once in spite of the Civil War. Kit Carson, the famous scout, was appointed to subdue the Navajo. Colonel Carson never had more than seven hundred men under his command and he had to face a nation of over ten thousand. His campaign in 1863 lasted less than twelve months, and although he never killed more than fifty Navajo, he was completely successful in destroying the nation. The Indians had been brought up with one idea of terror and brutality, the whites with another. Carson gave twenty-dollar bounties for every horse or mule either captured or killed and one-dollar bounties for sheep. All the enemies of the Navajo enthusiastically took part in the slaughter. Carson himself methodically destroyed all the crops he could find. In one canyon where Navajo sometimes hid, he spent several days making certain that three thousand peach trees were destroyed. At another place he captured seventy-five thousand pounds of wheat. At still another spot, the land itself was burned to prevent reseeding. Carson made total war in a manner the Indians had never imagined. The hungry and shocked Navajo began to surrender by the hundreds and then by the thousands.

In a sad trek of three hundred miles which the Navajo have called the Long Walk, they were forced to move to a barren spot in New Mexico called the *Bosque Redondo*. A new fort was constructed in the area to police the bands and prevent escapes. The brutalities and deaths of the forced march to the distant sickly place were as horrible and as needless as the suffering the Cherokee had experienced in 1838 on their Trail of Tears, when they had been forced at gunpoint to move from the Carolinas to Oklahoma. The Navajo were sheepless, seedless, and hopeless. They languished for five heartbreaking years, learning nothing and barely surviving. Their pleas to have a reservation in their old territories were not met until they took a sacred oath that they would never raid again. It was a pledge they made and kept. Manuelito, an important Navajo chief, remembered the day the Navajo returned to their homeland. "We told the drivers to whip the mules, we were in such a hurry. When we saw the top of the mountain from Albuquerque we wondered if it was our mountain and we felt like talking to the ground we loved it so, and some of the old men and women cried with joy . . ."

The Navajo received some seeds for their new reservation land, and by 1869 some of them began to work with silver, a craft which would one day help lift some of them to relative financial security. But life was an unending trial during the first bitter years of reservation existence. There was continual trouble about cattle. Many tribesmen lived a few miles off the actual reservation and this created difficulties with the whites, although the reservations were eventually expanded to take in the already de facto Navajo land. Treacherous agents tricked them systematically. Traders exploited them as a matter of routine. The Indian Bureau methodically attempted to destroy every traditional custom. Fifteen years passed before the tools and wagons promised to them were delivered. The weather was terrible and the crops failed. There were never-ending delays in getting needed lands and tools. Many individuals lapsed into alcoholism, and the nation might have been overcome by the despondency that crippled so many tribes but for the women. Navajo women had always had an important place in tribal life. They had owned the sheep and had always had an equal voice in business matters. Now these resourceful and confident women put their en-

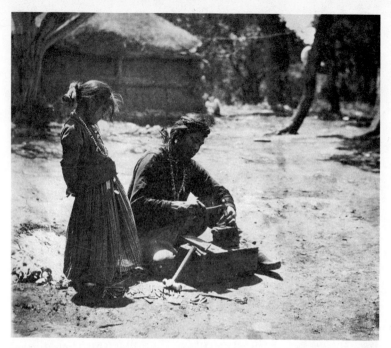

The work of silversmiths helped the Navajo to make a transition from their traditional way of life to life on the reservation. (*Courtesy of Museum of the American Indian, Heye Foundation*)

ergy into the art of weaving. Their rugs and blankets were done with such extraordinary skill that their fame quickly spread beyond the Southwest throughout the nation and even beyond both oceans.

In the slowest most painful sort of way, the earnings from silverwork and weaving allowed the tribe to grow. Sheep were bought and agricultural techniques mastered. The Navajo were the Great Learners and, at last, they found a way to live within the white man's framework. As the tribes around them grew poorer, the Navajo prospered. Once the Pueblo had dominated the region and the Navajo had been marauding outsiders. By mid-twentieth century the Navajo had become the largest and wealthiest tribe in the United States. But even in the midst of their success, there were Navajo who starved because there were many bands who fell into the pattern of the Pima and Papago. Their silverwork was not for their own pleasure and use but was a commodity to be sold as their weaving and admission to their sacred ceremonies were sold. Once there had been a time when the Navajo were poor, but they had all been poor together. Once there had been a time when the Navajo were rich, and they had all been rich together. Under the new system there were Navajo who held a million United States dollars and there were Navajo who died of malnutrition and starvation.

The traditional Navajo religion taught that the sun and the moon were bright shields carried by immortal beings on horseback. Such ideas were eventually mingled with Christian teachings but Navajo sand paintings remained as they had always been: the artist sits in the open or in a small hut and makes patterns with sand to guarantee the harmony of the universe. The colored sand is so skillfully sifted that true lines can be drawn as easily as circles and intricate configurations. The red, yellow, and black earth colors generally follow the pattern of a pair of lines in the center crossing at right angles upon which stand tall humanlike figures wearing masks. Many colored lines blend into the pattern to form reptiles, rainbows, and other natural elements. The paintings vary greatly in form and content, but their precision speaks of their importance. As the sand painter works, the Navajo live again. The history and the wisdom of the Navajo once more are released into the cosmos. The artist expresses his proud respect for all the natural phenomena, and when his design is done, he must smudge it out, for all life is temporary. Each hand makes a subtle variation in the most ancient design, but however full of joy and sorrow and struggle and beauty the design of any one day may be, it, too, will surely pass away just as in

the new year, another hand will create yet another variation.

THE RAIDERS

Perhaps no tribe has been so maligned as the Apache.
Partially this has to do with the nature of the tribe and partially because the Apache were among the last Indians to
threaten the security of the United States. They came to
the Southwest at the same time as the Navajo but unlike
them, the Apache preferred to remain raiders and were
never greatly influenced by Pueblo or Spanish ways. The
Apache fought for property, not glory. They counted no
coups and celebrated no scalp-taking. Those, who fought
them rarely even saw them, for the Apache were the mas-
ters of camouflage and swift movement, able to vanish into
the barren desert or mountains, to move faster on foot than
pursuing cavalry on horses. They wore no feather head-
dresses for dime novelists to write glowing paragraphs
about, and they valued the horse more for its food value
than for beauty or transportation.

If there was little about the Apache to romanticize, they
were still far from the heartless savages their enemies often
made them out to be. The Apache roamed in small bands
and one of the primary attributes of a leader was that he
must not lose many warriors. A cousin of Geronimo has
left a valuable record of that warrior's raiding and he states
that life was held in such high regard that a victory dance
would frequently be omitted if one of the band had been
killed. Likewise the most important religious, aesthetic,
and social event of the Apache had nothing to do with war

or the military arts but concerned females at puberty. At this time the girl became White Painted Lady (mother earth) and complicated ceremonies retold the creation myths and took the girl through all the stages of her future life. Individuals who assisted a family at this ritual became as close to one another as mortal can be to mortal. Even in the midst of marauding and eluding U.S. cavalry, Geronimo's band always allowed for the puberty rituals.

Such regard for women and for the life of their fellow tribesmen was among the finest traits of the Apache. They thought peace in the heart was the principal virtue. Should a woman be captured on a raid, a man was not to have her unless he first opened her heart and won her through love. The Apache had hundreds of songs for this and similar purposes. Apache girls have written that people would fall in love by the campfires just by listening to songs. These melodies were often short and direct yet all the more charming and sensitive for their naïve frankness,

> My sweetheart, we surely could have gone home.
> But you were afraid!
> When it was night, we surely could have gone home.
> But you were afraid!

The Apache generally took no adult male prisoners unless they were to be sold as slaves, but children, especially boys, were often treated as natural offspring. They were taught that the highest virtues were to speak the truth, to pay their debts, and never to steal from their own kind. Only then could an individual know peace of heart. Clan and marital loyalties were primary, making Apache camps places of wit and good cheer. The bands loved all social activities, gambling, and sports. Their fondness for drink became legendary and was a large part of social life both on the reservations and off. They were constantly on the move and had no time to produce objects of beauty, yet like all peoples the Apache character had many levels. The killer raider of the trail was the joking lover of the campsite. He was also the one who taught children how to capture delicate butterflies and then release them without harm.

The bands liked to establish mountain strongholds from which to attack the neighboring pueblos and Mexican land. Apache women planted gardens of corn, beans, and squash, as well as harvesting cactus fruit. Their main staple was a meal made of corn and mesquite beans which had the double advantage of being easy to grow and light to carry. The principal source of wealth, however, was stolen property. Though the Apache disliked routine work and restraint of any kind, they had the patience to plan and execute complex ambushes. The Apache military strategy outwitted some of the best generals of West Point and many plans were co-ordinated over large areas even though the tribe operated in widely scattered units that were extremely jealous of their individual rights and independence.

The history of any given Apache group is almost impossible to trace because of certain taboos and because of the lack of written records. One of these taboos was that if an individual died, his name must not be repeated. The deeds of great warriors were thus quickly forgotten, but even more damage was done to the work of future historians if the man's name coincided with that of a common bird or animal, which was often the case. If the name of the dead man were Bald Eagle, the band would have to devise a new way of saying *bald* and *eagle*. The language was thus constantly changing. The grandmother in a family might not always be able to communicate with her grandchildren. Another taboo was that Apache must never eat creatures that lived in water. Likewise, although they hunted for the feathers of certain birds, many of the same birds were taboo as far as eating was concerned. Apache fear of the dead cannot be too much exaggerated. They liked to bury the deceased in daylight, if possible on the very day of death, and then immediately to cleanse themselves for fear of contamination. Their fear of the dead led to a terror of owls, whose voices were the song of death. A hooting owl in the night could frighten them as no human sound ever could.

While the various name taboos and fears of the dead have blotted much of Apache history, like most Indians the Apache had excellent memories. Many historians have noted that the memories of old people among the Sioux and Apache are more accurate than the written accounts of whites. Jason Betzinez, the cousin of Geronimo, broke many of the Apache taboos in his writing. As a teen-ager Betzinez fought with bow and arrow in a Stone Age struggle against the cavalry yet he lived to hear the blast of the atom and watch the flaming tails of guided missiles in the very same desert. This intriguing figure wrote of the Indian oral tradition,

> To the Indian it is a curious thing that white people accept as fact only that which is written on paper, whereas events retold by word of mouth, even if of greater importance, are disparaged as being mere folklore.

The relationship between the Apache and the Mexicans was so bitter that the Apache tended to trust the United States more than most Indians did. Nevertheless when the bluecoats arrived in force to put the Apache on reservations, the various bands resisted. The details of the army-Apache struggles are the familiar ones except for one unique episode. That exception concerns Cochise, one of the most able of the Chiricahua chiefs, and Tom Jeffords, a white adventurer. Cochise was a handsome man but like all Apache, when he painted his face to lead a group of shouting, excited, armed raiders, he looked fierce. Cochise explained Apache ways with these words:

> God made us not as you; we were born like the animals, in the dry grass, not on beds like you. This is why we do as the animals, go about at night and rob and steal. If had such things as you have, I would not do as I do, for then I would not need to do so.

Apache fury, however, was not the cause of Cochise going to war with the whites. He had always been at peace with the United States until 1860 when a young officer tricked him into bringing his family to dine at an army camp. A boy had recently been stolen by some Indians and the officer intended to hold Cochise and his family as hostages. Cochise had had nothing to do with the kidnaping, so the plan would have failed even if the unarmed chief had not managed to escape. He soon secured white hostages of his own. The official army records state Cochise grew so irrational that he killed his hostages, which prompted the local officers to kill his family, a war crime under any circumstance. The Apache version seems more logical, especially given their well-known regard for the lives of their family and tribesmen. The Apache claimed they had taken the whites only to exchange them for their own people. When they neared the army camp, they discovered the army had already slain them. Only then did Cochise hang his hostages. He chose the same tree where his own people had been slain. The war that followed was merciless. A sergeant sympathetic to Cochise and a supporter of the Apache version of the incident said that during that spring alone, Cochise personally burned alive thirteen whites, tortured five others by cutting pieces out of their bodies, and dragged fifteen others to death after tying a lariat around their necks. The sergeant commented sadly, "This Indian was at peace until betrayed and wounded by white men."

When the Civil War caused the Union to withdraw many troops for battles in the East, the Apache, like other Indians in the West, thought their resistance had finally weakened the whites. When various units of Confederate and Union troops appeared in the area, the Apache attacked them vigorously, hoping to drive out the divided white tribes completely. Different bands under various head men such as Cochise fought under the general but loose leadership of Magnas Coloradas, a war chief who proved to be an elusive enemy for the whites. Massacres, cruelty, and treachery on the part of whites and Apache alike during this period surpass the ferocity of anything previously experienced in the wars with Indians. At last the army sent a messenger to Magnas Coloradas in 1863, guaranteeing him safe conduct if he came to talk peace. When the chief accepted, he was captured, tortured, and "shot while trying to escape."

Cochise and his two thousand Chiricahua continued to struggle. Eventually they took possession of an impregnable mountain area they called the Stronghold. Campaigns to take Cochise were futile, but by 1872 the aging chief hoped to establish a permanent peace for his people. Tom Jeffords, a tall athletic man whom the Indians called Red Beard, proved to be the key figure in the settlement. He had had the respect and friendship of the Chiricahua ever since he had had the courage to come to the Stronghold unarmed to bargain a right of way for a stagecoach line. Now, Jeffords wanted to bring General Howard into the Stronghold for a peace parley.

When the two chiefs met, the general promised Cochise a large reservation some miles distant where all the Apache bands could be together. Cochise refused Howard's offer because he did not think the various Apache could live in peace with each other. Furthermore, he knew the army would never be able to control American civilians even if it wanted to, any more than he could control his own hotter bloods. Without the Stronghold, the Chiricahua would surely perish. Nevertheless he called in all his captains for their opinions. They decided that a reservation was acceptable, provided it was the Stronghold they now ruled. With their many well-armed braves under their own leaders in places they had known since birth, they could resist vastly superior forces. Even the very rocks were good friends who would protect them from bullets. Howard hesitated about letting Cochise have the Stronghold but the chief insisted, just as he insisted that Jeffords must be his agent, an honor Jeffords would just as soon have declined. The army was skeptical about Howard's bargain but decided to go along and the war arrows were broken.

Jeffords was an army captain at the time of the signing but the Apache were less impressed by his rank than by his genuine sense of justice. His dealings with the Chiricahua were always honorable and as long as Cochise lived there was no more fighting. Jeffords was under no illusions regarding the Apache character. He knew Cochise drank too much. He knew the chief sometimes beat his wives. He understood that Cochise was the same mixture of good and evil that all men are. The image of the blood-savoring savage was quite as false as that of the denatured, desexed Noble Savage of the missionaries and idealistic philosophers.

Just a few months before his death, Cochise had mellowed to a point where he allowed Mexicans to cross his reservation to trade, but he forbade them to cross with weapons as they had done on an earlier illegal trip. Cochise ordered rather than begged. He spoke with the authority earned as head man of the council of the Chiricahua Apache and he died exercising the full democratic power of his responsible position. The night before his death, Cochise sent for Jeffords. The old chief wanted a farewell talk with his younger friend. General Howard himself had stated that Cochise deployed men as skillfully as any officer the general had ever seen. But now, knowing that he was about to die, the chief's thoughts were on other matters. The Indians rarely quarreled about religion and each man thought of the hereafter in his own terms. Cochise said he had been dwelling on the problem of death and he had decided that an afterlife existed and that Jeffords would be there to share it with him. The categories of Indian and non-Indian were erased that night as two men talked of the ancient mysteries by the light of burning wood. The sympathy that bound them was something that could have arisen between their nations. The Indian often demonstrated he was ready to ride such a trail but the whites shunned such a road from their first steps upon what they arrogantly called a virgin continent. They continued to shun the road until long after they had finally succeeded in placing every red tribe upon a reservation.

Of the many commanders who fought against them, the Apache respected General Crook above all others. He had come to command in 1872 after a treacherous massacre of the Apache at Camp Grant the year before. Crook was an unspectacular soldier who employed basic strategy with a concern for each particular situation. His first preparation for fighting the Apache was to train small mobile columns supplied with the best mule trains available. Crook also made it a practice to hire Indian scouts and during his year in the Southwest he employed some five hundred Apache at the same pay as regular soldiers. The Apache were allowed their own war leaders who served as sergeants. These were often the best units to use against rival bands of Apache. The policy of making Apache warriors soldiers was obviously more sensible than trying to force them to be farmers, but the Indian Bureau wanted to have all Indians on reservations and it wanted all reservation Indians to be farmers.

Crook's success among the Apache led him to be promoted to commander of the entire region surrounding the Platte River in the North. As soon as Crook departed from Apache country, a foolish policy was adopted which concentrated all the Apache upon a few dry and cheerless reservations. Often groups more hostile to each other than to whites were placed on the same reservation. The situation could only result in new rebellions, and when they occurred they were as fierce as the ones Crook had helped to end. The new Apache head man was Victorio, whose band of never more than one hundred warriors killed one hundred United States soldiers, two hundred United States civilians, and two hundred Mexicans. Victorio campaigned from 1877–80 before being killed by Mexicans.

Reservation life would have been difficult for the Apache under any circumstance, but the Indian Bureau seemed to go out of its way to create trouble. The Department of the Interior had been created in 1849 and the Indian Bureau had been transferred to it from the War Department, although the War Department also continued to have power to deal with the Indians. After 1879, the Indian Bureau adopted a rigid policy of destroying everything that was distinctly Indian, especially Indian religion, language, and social habits. On many occasions, high-ranking military officers in actual contact with Indians had a better appreciation and sensitivity for their culture than the civilians of the Indian Bureau. The civilians tended to have special interests regarding Indians. They sometimes wanted to convert them to specific Christian churches and quite often they simply wanted to cheat them of supplies and land.

The Apache got particularly bad treatment because of their reputations as incorrigible fighters. No livestock was delivered to them. No effort was made to employ them in the manner Crook had. Tribes who had feuds with one another had to share the same land. Various groups were shuffled from place to place without their consent and without any apparent reason. Victorio's break was seen as inevitable, and, as the inevitable will, it happened again and again. The new rebels were motivated by two things: they wanted to live the exciting life of the past and they feared the whites would kill them during their periodic fits of violence. The most important of the new rebels was Geronimo, a warrior who had fought under Magnas Colorados and Cochise.

Geronimo's legend is spectacular, but his exploits were neither high-minded nor inspiring. He was not a Pontiac or a Tecumseh with a vision of uniting the Indians. Geronimo was simply a marauder, a marauder of the sort the Apache had always been. He was concerned with keeping his band as safe and prosperous as possible. He was neither more nor less cruel, more nor less cunning, more nor less set in his ways than most other Apache head men. Like other bands, his men knew the land so well that a few stones out of place would give them important information. They were able to walk seventy-five miles a day in the hottest deserts. They signaled to each other with sudden puffs of smoke in graceful clouds to let their comrades know strange parties were approaching. Rapidly multiplying clouds meant the travelers were well armed, and steady smoke meant the band should collect at some prearranged place for joint action. At night the flames of a fire set on a high mesa could be used the same way.

The campaigns of Geronimo were filled with murder, but the treachery he had personally experienced was rarely mentioned by his white enemies. Geronimo had lost his mother, his wife, and three children in an unprovoked Mexican raid. He knew that almost two hundred Apache women and children had been killed at the Camp Grant Massacre. He knew that an army officer had cut off the head of Magnas Colorados and sent it east as a curiosity. He knew how the war with Cochise had begun. He always claimed that the reason he left the reservations so many times was that the whites were always threatening to jail or kill him.

General Crook was called to Apache country in 1882 in hopes that he could renew his successes against the Indians. His first move was to organize a new corps of scouts. Within a short time, he was able to cross into Mexico and enter the Sierre Madre camp of Geronimo. The talk between the two chiefs went well. Geronimo agreed to return to the San Carlos reservation once he gathered up his scattered families. Some Apache returned immediately with Crook, and weeks later Geronimo himself turned up with a stolen herd of cattle of over three hundred head. Crook was severely criticized for his handling of the wily Geronimo by government officials who wanted quick decisive defeats. They did not understand Geronimo was acting in the proper Apache fashion in providing his people with cattle, just as Geronimo did not understand why Crook took away those cattle. The officials also did not understand that Crook's honorable manner of dealing with Apache was the best if not the only way to prevent new outbreaks.

There is good evidence that Geronimo tried to be a farmer after his first surrender to Crook. Unfortunately, the newspapers played up his former raids in sensational stories. Dishonest political forces in Tucson were anxious for more Indian trouble, and there was continual arguing over policy between the army and the Indian Bureau. By the spring of 1885 the tensions on Geronimo became too great for him to bear. In later years, he would explain the cause of his outbreak:

> I was living peaceably with my family, having plenty to eat, sleeping well, taking care of my people, perfectly contented. I don't know where those bad stories first came from. There we were, doing well and being well. I was behaving well. I hadn't killed a horse or a man, American or Indian. I don't know what was the matter with the people in charge of us. They knew this to be so, and yet they said I was a bad man and the worst man there; but what harm had I done? I was living peaceably and well, but I did not leave on my own accord. Had I left it would have been right to blame me; but as it is, blame those men who started this talk about me.

What followed was a year and a half of violent marauding, sometimes with luck, sometimes with hard times, but always with death. The size of the band was never the same, the braves came and left whenever they wished. The Mexicans and Americans pursued with great determination, but Geronimo might have stayed out indefinitely had not many of his people become lonesome for their relatives at San Carlos. One of his half brothers wanted to surrender in order to be with his wife again. Other brothers said they did not want him to go in alone.

A peace was almost accomplished about a year after the outbreak. General Crook again managed to get word to

Geronimo about a peace conference. The two leaders, accompanied by their warriors, met at Canyon de los Embudos in northern Mexico from March 25 to March 27. A photographer took pictures so that "the folks back East" could see what the mighty Geronimo looked like. The chief agreed to return to San Carlos but that very night a smuggler sold him liquor and Geronimo bolted with a third of his band, leaving seventy-seven Apache to be taken as prisoners of war.

Crook was again criticized for his handling of the matter and he asked to be relieved of his command. His successor was General Miles who was ordered to pursue and destroy the hostile Indians while making maximum use of regular troops. This direct policy statement implied criticism of the use of Apache scouts, who some bureaucrats thought were in league with Geronimo. Miles had an additional two thousand men assigned to him, bringing his command to a full five thousand soldiers. Miles also had use of the heliograph, a new wireless telegraphic device involving mirrors. This gadget had just been perfected by the signal corps to co-ordinate the movement of troops over wide areas. The general campaigned with all his energy and skill but during four vigorous months in the field, neither he, nor his heliographic corps, nor his five thousand men could kill or capture a single Apache.

When word arrived that Geronimo was again willing to negotiate, Miles sent a lieutenant and two Apache scouts to investigate. Geronimo was being hard pressed by the Mexicans and wanted to surrender to the United States. His band had been fluctuating as usual. His top strength had been thirty-five warriors with about one hundred women and children. When he actually surrendered he had two dozen men and fourteen women and children with him. During his time off the reservation he had only lost six men and four women while killing ten bluecoats, twelve Indian scouts, seventy-five United States civilians, and one hundred Mexicans.

Geronimo's surrender in September 1886 was turned into a catastrophe for the entire Chiricahua people for they were all shipped to Florida as incorrigible prisoners of war. All the Chiricahua were sent whether they had remained on the reservation or had fought, whether they were warriors, old men, women, or infants. Even the two scouts who had risked their lives to arrange the surrender were imprisoned. The racist assumptions behind Indian policy had never been so blatantly exposed. The toll in

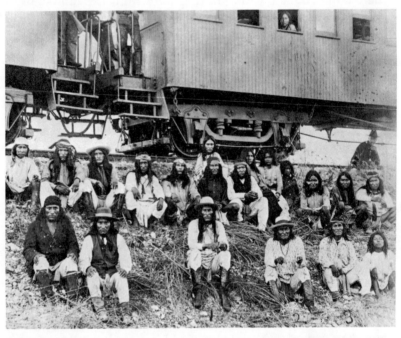

The legendary Geronimo is third from the right in the front row of these Apache prisoners being shipped to Florida by train. (*National Archives*)

sickness and death took its place beside the Cherokee Trail of Tears and the Navajo Long Walk.

The Apache were kept in Florida until 1894 when they were transferred to Oklahoma where they were kept under guard until 1914. Geronimo survived the various movings and diseases and proved to be far less incorrigible than the Indian haters had claimed. He eventually took part in the inaugural parade of President Theodore Roosevelt and was a charmer who sold his autograph at regional and world fairs. The tough raider who had terrorized Americans and Mexicans for forty years even converted to Christianity, joining the Dutch Reformed Church in 1903. Geronimo had always been a heavy drinker, and it was the white man's whiskey which finally ended his life. One night while riding back from town in a drunken stupor, the eighty-year-old Geronimo fell from his seat and cracked open his skull upon his own wagon.

The Apache were as wild as the Pueblo were mystical, but their wildness partly sprang from an unrestrained love of personal freedom. The tale of Massai exhibits Apache exuberance at its best. He was a warrior who had fought with Geronimo at times and lived on a reservation at other times. When the Chiricahua were being packed into box-cars for shipment to Florida he urged a final uprising. Failing to convince the others, he sat quietly until one night in the middle of Kansas he jumped from the train. He had no idea of where he was. He could only travel at night. He could ask no one for help or directions. But he found his way back to the very place where he was born. Soon he stole a Mescalero woman and took her with him to the mountains where he lived another twenty-five years in absolute freedom.

The same spirit infused a handful of Chiricahua and

some San Carlos Apache who had not come in with Geronimo but stayed in Old Mexico as a distinct group until at
least the 1930s. Geronimo's cousin became a Presbyterian
and eagerly took up the ways of the whites, but he always
defended his people. He knew full well the contrast between the way Indians treated one another and the way
whites treated one another. He warned his white fellow
citizens:

> You white people can now go about your business
> without fear of attack by Apaches. But you are still
> subject to being preyed upon. Beware of your own
> race, who are seeking an easy path to wealth at your
> expense.

Part II

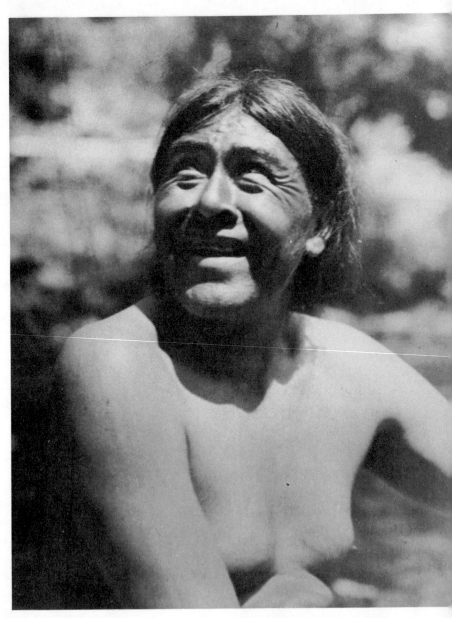

Ishi, last of the Yahi Indians of California. (*Lowie Museum of Anthropology, University of California, Berkeley*)

Where the Sun Falls into the Sea:
CALIFORNIA

You stay, I go

Epitaph of Ishi, Last of the Yahi

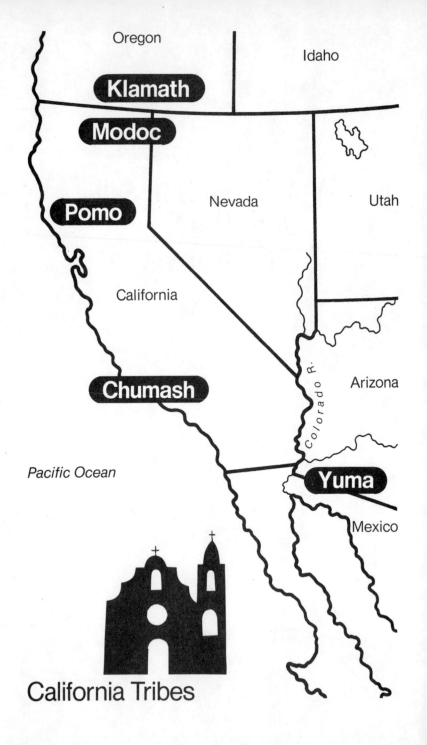

Oregon

Idaho

Klamath

Modoc

Nevada

Utah

Pomo

California

Colorado R.

Arizona

Chumash

Pacific Ocean

Yuma

Mexico

California Tribes

DEATH IN THE MISSIONS

California was the golden temptress of the frontier where the worst and best aspects of the West mingled freely like so many drinkers at a common bar. Even before the whites came, the area had been a mixture of different tribes living in patterns unlike the tribes of the Atlantic coast. The land was so bountiful that almost every migratory group passing through had left some part of its people to settle permanently. There were forty major groups speaking at least twenty languages with five hundred smaller divisions having a hundred dialects. At the time of the Spanish conquest over a hundred and fifty thousand Indians lived in California, making it one of the most densely populated regions in all of North America. Food was so abundant and the climate so favorable that loosely organized tribes had little experience with wars, social unrest, or deprivations. They were little given to fighting in any form and rarely moved from their traditional gathering grounds. Hospitality was their personal and national rule. Material wealth was accumulated for the pleasure of giving. Mystic religions and poetic rituals provided a rich ceremonial life from birth to death.

The Californians were simple people. Early travelers reported that they were birdlike even to their twittering speech and the bright colors with which they painted their bodies and possessions. The first visitors were greeted by canoes of singing Indians who came to see the bearded men who wore metal. They danced and played music for the newcomers. They had no fear of the whites and did everything they knew to make the strangers happy.

The life ways of Californians were determined primarily by the excellent climate and the fertile soil of their region. Acorns which were ground to meal and several types of corn could be had for the gathering, and provided the base for any number of tasty dishes. Flour was made from bitter plums. Roots, berries, nuts, greens, currants, small game, and the inexhaustible bounty of the sea added variety to a tribe's feasting. Rabbits were particularly plentiful and whatever was not available locally could be obtained by trading over sea or land.

The Californians lived out of doors most of the time, moving from one favored gathering place to another while carefully observing rigid tribal boundaries. When they required shelter, the Indians dug a hole about two feet deep and erected a hut of bush and bark supported on crisscrossed poles. They walked barefoot and wore few if any clothes although they liked to tattoo and paint themselves extensively. Some women covered their entire upper bodies with fine lattice patterns that gave the illusion of an intricately woven garment. Shells and unusual rocks were used by both sexes to make necklaces, earrings, combs, and arm bands.

The tribelets gathered or fished in small groups under the leadership of a head man and his council. The leader usually had a sacred hut or carried a "magic bundle" consisting of skins or feathers of creatures he had seen in a vision or found near a place where he had had a vision. The leader was always a good singer who knew the creation myths from beginning to end and generally, he was an expert in the eagle dance. The chiefs had few civil decisions to make as there was little to quarrel about. Children were never punished and there were few crimes. The one act that aroused indignation and carried the death penalty was when an individual used up food that had been gathered for the use of all. Feasts and dances were common, with puberty a special time for males and females. The boys' elaborate initiation rites included the use of the dangerous Jimson weed which was supposed to help the youths secure visions. Marriage came in late adolescence and men with more than one wife were common. Divorce was a simple matter with the female returning to her parent's home and both parties easily securing new mates.

Strangely enough, the happy singers to whom so much had been given were the Indians who thought most about death. Their dead were cremated, and elaborate mourning procedures were required one year after the cremation. Some tribes placed the ashes of the dead in exquisite jars which rivaled their baskets in beauty and grace. The Yuma, who lived on the deserts bordering the Colorado River, developed the death phobia to its fullest degree. They did not have the elaborate rituals of the corn-growing pueblo dwellers. Rather than being concerned with the powers that control rain, Yuma creation myths were pessimistic and dealt with a dying god. Different versions of the myth had the god becoming the first cremation and his son or brother continuing the work of making the Colorado River and holy places. The California tribes tended to be less extreme in their beliefs, but they had the same basic viewpoint. In one legend, the god Wiyot knew his daughter would poison him. Each month he would ask, "Shall I die this month?"

The Spanish missionaries who established their first churches in 1769 sought to erase the death religions with their promise of resurrection, but they ended by playing the daughter to the Californian's Wiyot. Legends of a lost tribe of white brothers aided the padres in making their first converts as the Indians flocked to accept the magic of the gray robes and to marvel at the strength and beauty of the new places of worship. The Franciscans brought grapes, plums, olives, oranges, carrots, lettuce, and cabbage as well as new tools such as the plow, hoe, pick, and spade. The Indians were fascinated by all the new things but they soon discovered the Spanish would not allow them to live as they had in the past. The Indians were forced to settle within the mission walls, and soldiers made certain they did not run away. If an Indian attempted to escape, he was tracked down and punished severely. The Christian fathers had pledged lives of poverty and industry, but they made the Indians work hard to create the wealth that enabled the Franciscan order to extend its missions up the entire California coast. Indians worked that soldiers could be well fed and comfortable. Once they had been able to get all they needed by simply taking it from the earth. Now, they labored all day to earn a pint of corn.

Men and women who had always lived in freedom were locked in the mission compounds from nine in the evening until morning prayers. The people who had enjoyed nudity were forced to wear pants, skirts, shoes, and shirts. Any who dared rebel were whipped or placed in stocks or shackled. The Californians had never known punishment yet now their women might be locked in stocks for three days and their men lashed until blood ran down their backs. The Indians had been possessed with thoughts of death and now death became their constant, often welcomed, comrade. Mothers sometimes chose to smother their newborn rather than subject them to mission life.

When Mexico won independence from Spain all aid to the missions was cut off. The last mission was built in 1832 and two summers later economic collapse shattered the

Franciscan empire. The Indians had been wrenched from their traditional ways yet they had never been allowed to integrate into the new. Their hearts had long been broken and now their bodies could not resist the starvation, despondency, and diseases which swept the compounds. By 1880 there would be fewer than twenty thousand Indians in all of California and half of those would be reservation hostages from other states.

The missionaries were so zealous in spreading Catholicism that they ignored the ancient lore of the people they sought to convert. Rich Indian cultures passed into oblivion without any effort to preserve their languages, traditions, and religions. The ecological balance which had been developed over hundreds of years perished under the well-meaning but stern Franciscan heel. Even the economic collapse of 1834 would have been far less disastrous if the Indians had not already been psychologically destroyed. Their imaginative spirit and colorful life had been torn from them in a manner whose thoroughness was matched only by its speed. Only a single lifetime separated the ways of the centuries from the shattered refugees of the mission compounds. Californians were folk of the dance and song. They were the spontaneous, the unfettered. Disease, murder, exploitation, and economic depression destroyed them in a way unprecedented even in the United States.

The greed of the Gold Rush was the final seal on the Indian coffin. The padres had desired to help the Indians, the miners of 1849 wished only to destroy them. The U. S. Government encouraged rather than restrained its citizens in their Indian hatred. During the first years of the 1850s, treaties were negotiated with hundreds of tribes residing in the best parts of the state. The agreements deprived the Indians of almost all their lands, but still the California whites thought the treaties were much too generous. Their representatives in Washington were so powerful that the United States Senate refused to ratify the treaties. The Indian Bureau had never been noted for its integrity and after the political death of the treaties, the bureau lived up to its bad reputation by consciously adopting a policy of open deception. The bureau simply failed to inform the Indians that the treaties had been rejected by the Great Council of the whites. The honest tribesmen abided by their agreements only to have the white government sell every acre of land promised to them.

Little is known of the cultures that were snuffed out so quickly. The objects that do survive suggest that the Californians may have been among the most interesting of all the Indian nations, certainly the most delightful. The women of the Pomo in central California were so skillful at weaving that a microscope is needed to see their individual stitches. Colored designs were improved by working in the brilliant feathers of birds such as woodpeckers and warblers. The birds also influenced Californian music. The most common instruments aside from the human voice were wooden whistles and rattles made of shells and pebbles. Music was almost always accompanied by singing or dancing. Among some tribes the shamans performed a fire dance in which they pushed hot embers into a pile with their bare feet.

California art achieved its most individual tone in a small area around what is now Santa Barbara, where a tribe called the Chumash lived. The Chumash have left eighty sites of distinctive rock paintings. Their work is not drawn lifelike, but highly stylized and semiabstract. Buglike creatures with angular bodies serve as the main features. Black, red, and white coloring predominate with an occasional sprinkling of yellow. A marvelous sense of humor and liberty infuses every line. The delightful animals have

multiple legs, pinwheel heads, and tails that look like ex-
ploding fireworks. The paintings range from being several
inches long to huge efforts covering more than forty feet
of cave wall. Some are simple line drawings and others
are full paintings. They were pecked, cut, and rubbed
on cavern walls. The Chumash loved to paint whatever
they could—their faces, their bodies, their weapons, their
few clothes. Their canoes were bathed in red and colored
boards marked their burial places. The joyful rock paintings inspire the viewer to know more of the people who
made them. But there is no one left to speak of them. The
California tribes were too gentle to survive white civilization. They were like the eagle of one of their myths who
sang:

> At the time of death
> when I found there was to be death,
> I was very much surprised.
> All was failing.
> My home,
> I was sad to leave it.
>
> I have been looking far,
> sending my spirit north, south, east, and west
> trying to escape death
> but could find nothing.
> No way to escape.

CAPTAIN JACK

Few of the Californians knew how to fight back against
the whites, but one small group humiliated the United
States army in a fashion unique in the Indian wars. In a

struggle lasting almost half a year a handful of poorly equipped Modoc warriors held off an entire army. Their successes indicate how much damage the Indians might have done had their notions of war and honor been different than they were.

The Modoc bands had done some raiding and fighting in the 1850s but the whites had retaliated with so many soldiers and massacres that the tribe had agreed to a reservation. They took up the white man's clothing and habits, and they tried to live in peace. The only other Indians who spoke the same language happened to be the Klamath, who lived just north of them in Oregon. In its usual disregard for Indian feuds, the Indian Bureau placed the Modoc and Klamath on the same reservation. The inevitable quarrels broke out and several Modoc groups left the reservation to return to their old homes along Lost River.

On November 28, 1872, thirty-eight soldiers were dispatched to bring in the band of Kintpuash (known to the whites as Captain Jack because of his fondness for bits and pieces of military uniforms and paraphernalia). The Modoc had not left the reservation on a whim and they resisted the troops sent to take them back. The soldiers retreated to get reinforcements and the band headed for a place they called Land-of-Burnt-out-Fires, an area of lava beds. The wild jumble of caverns and ridges made the land look like a hard sponge. One section called the Stronghold was surrounded by chasms that formed natural trench systems, which made the higher ground like a fortified castle. A few parts of the lava beds were fertile and provided enough water and game for the small band of perhaps 120 Modoc. Within a short time an additional group from Hot Creek under the leadership of Curly Headed Doctor and Hooker Jim joined the band of Captain Jack. The total

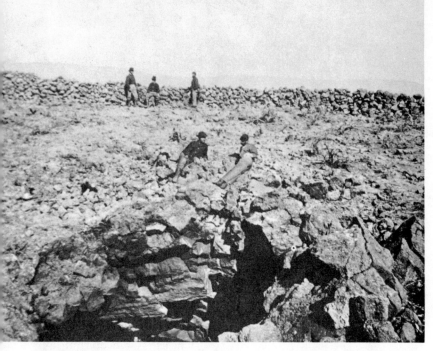

From caves such as this one in the middle of rugged lava beds, the
Modoc followers of Captain Jack were able to hold off U.S. soldiers
for months. (*National Archives*)

combined warrior strength was never more than fifty but
the fortresslike terrain gave the Modoc strength far beyond
their numbers.

A large body of troops arrived at the lava beds in early
January. The soldiers attempted to assault the Modoc
positions in a traditional frontal attack, but the Indians
had learned every twist of every ridge and had prepared
special vantage points for their fighting men. White casualties mounted at a rapid rate with no Modoc being seen,
much less injured or captured. Bullets and howitzer shells
uselessly ricocheted off rocks and were more dangerous
to those who fired them than to their Modoc targets. The
Indians were made even more confident when they saw

that no soldier was able to pass beyond the magic line drawn by Curly Headed Doctor.

Repeated attempts to take the lava beds were equally futile, and the army sent word that it wanted to negotiate. Captain Jack was willing to take a reservation as long as it was separate from the Klamath, but men like Hooker Jim and Curly Headed Doctor had other fears. They had committed crimes of robbery and murder and thought the whites would punish them if they surrendered. Captain Jack stated his dilemma as chief of the rebels:

> I want to go and see my people on the reservation. My mind is made up to say "yes." I have a good heart, and want no mistake made this time, to live with good heart and talk truth. I have no paper men, and can't write on paper. The papers called me bad and lied about me. If they don't lie to me, I won't lie to them. I want to give up shooting . . . I wish to live like the whites. Let everything be wiped out, washed out, and let there be no more blood. I have got a bad heart about those murderers. I have got but a few men and I don't see how I can give them up. Will they give up their people who murdered my people while they were asleep? . . . I can see how I could give up my horse to be hanged; but I can't see how I could give up my men to be hanged. I could give up my horse to be hanged and I wouldn't cry about it; but if I gave up my men I would have to cry about it. I want them all to have good hearts now. I have thrown everything away. There must be no more bad talk. I will not. I have spoken forever. I want soldiers all to go home. I have given up now and want no more fuss. I have said yes and thrown away my country. I want soldiers to go away so I will not be afraid.

The one thing that was certain was that the soldiers

would not go away. Their defeat had not affected their confidence but it had injured their pride. A peace commission began to meet with the Modoc leaders in February. Its leadership soon fell to Brigadier General Canby, commander of the entire region. The Modoc retained their strong military positions and their previous victories meant they were able to bargain from strength. They were amazed and insulted to discover the army came not to discuss but to dictate. Canby presented a series of demands. Jack was annoyed. "I will not agree on anything you may offer until you agree to give me a home in my native country." Jack asked for a specific place long wanted as a reservation by the Modoc but he said his men might settle for the lava beds to show their reasonableness. The army responded that it couldn't take up the matter of a reservation, that reservations were civilian, not military matters. Canby even pressed the Modoc leadership on the question of unpunished criminals who were fighting with Jack. The chief again answered that he was willing to give up his accused men for white trial whatever day the whites chose to give up their men who were accused of murdering Modoc women for Indian trial. Reverend Thomas, another member of the negotiating commission, told Jack that he must place more trust in God. Jack countered that he trusted the spirits very much but that unfortunately he was not dealing with the spirits but with soldiers wearing blue cloth and brass buttons.

The bargaining dragged on for more than two months. The Modoc grew more and more impatient with Jack, and the government pressed Canby to make some agreement or resume the fighting. Some of Jack's men said he was a coward. Others accused him of wanting to betray them for personal gain. Curly Headed Doctor suggested

Jack could prove his bravery by killing everyone on the peace commission at a meeting. During the heat of one debate, several friends of Curly Headed Doctor snuck up behind Jack and placed a woman's headdress and female garments on him. Jack tore away the clothes angrily and shouted that if there was to be any killing he would slay Canby himself. Later he asked the council to release him from his oath. "Death is mighty bad. Death will come to us soon enough." His men would not reverse their decision and Jack agreed to go through with the pledge rather than lose leadership of the group.

At the new conference, Captain Jack repeated his position and Canby repeated his. As no compromise seemed possible Jack kept the promise he had given his followers and shot General Canby beneath the right eye. The commissioner who had wanted the Modoc to place more trust in God was also shot. Other warriors set upon two other commissioners but a Modoc woman had given them advance warning of possible trouble and the alerted men were able to escape with minor wounds. After returning to his stronghold, Jack's original doubts about the wisdom of the killings returned. He spent much of his time meditating in the cave which he used as his home.

Canby was the highest-ranking officer ever to be killed by Indians, but, of course, his murder could not possibly aid the Modoc cause. The Indians thought that killing the leader of the besieging forces would make them headless warriors who would lose heart and go home. They did not realize that the United States army had a hundred generals and that the pony soldiers were not Indians who fought according to individual will but paid fighters who were drilled in the strictest discipline.

The shocked and angered soldiers grouped their forces to deal the Modoc a blow that would wipe them out.

Four companies of reserves were brought to the lava beds, bringing a section of twelve-pound mortars and men who could handle the weapons with better skill than the cavalrymen had. From their vantage points, eight Indians had been able to pin down four hundred soldiers. The shells had rebounded harmlessly on rocks and the magic rope of Curly Headed Doctor had not been crossed. In the new fighting the Modoc did not fare as well. The army attacked in two strong columns supported by heavy mortar and howitzer fire. They were able to gain territory and cut off the Modoc from their supply of water. The army clearly won the battle, but all the members of the band escaped capture.

The months that followed were a cycle of hide-and-seek fighting in the rocks. The army was tireless in its searching but the Modoc were just as untiring in eluding. The Modoc relied heavily on ambushes and attacking dozing sentries. They sometimes raided ranches in the area and ran off livestock for food. A typical fight occurred on April 6 when twenty-one soldiers were killed and twenty more wounded in an ambush. Even more might have died if a relief column had not been attracted by the shooting. The soldiers grew so desperate that when they found one dead Modoc warrior, they cut his scalp into a hundred pieces and even shaved off his eyebrows.

The only chance the band had was to exhaust the soldiers. They might have succeeded if arguments had not begun to split them. Curly Headed Doctor sought to convince Jack's men to fight under his leadership, but they stayed loyal to their original head man. The fourteen warriors following the medicine man often fought independently of Jack's men. At least three hundred soldiers were always in the field against the Modoc. In early May the Modoc prepared a new ambush by Dry Lake, an area of volcanic ashes. The army horses were successfully stampeded but a charge on foot broke the Modoc force into small parties. Curly Headed Doctor, Hooker Jim, and others were captured. They offered to scout against Jack if they would be shown clemency for the crimes they had committed before the outbreak of the miniature war. The army agreed for, as long as Jack was free, the Modoc would continue to fight. The individual who had been taunted for being a coward proved to have the strongest will and bravest spirit while his tormentors became traitors. When the turncoats approached Jack about surrendering, he spat out his defiance and refused to talk with them. Some of Jack's followers talked for a time with the turncoats but no agreement was possible. A few of the Modoc families slipped back to the reservation making a *de facto* peace of their own. Jack regretted the killing of Canby, and the life of constant war oppressed his spirit. Food was scarce and water was particularly difficult to get. Life had become an endless hunt with Jack the chief prey. Hooker Jim and others led the army to where Jack was camped. He might have escaped but Modoc disunity and the idea of once more fleeing at last broke him. His statement upon surrender was blunt. "My legs have given out."

The members of the band were treated as prisoners of war, but the six individuals who were responsible for the actual murdering of the peace commissioners were held as criminals. A trial was convened under the white man's law and the death verdict duly arrived at. Jack's good humor and no nonsense attitude stayed with him to the end. When he was told by a well-meaning minister that he was going to a better place than anything on earth, Jack offered the minister the privilege of taking his place. He added he would throw in all his horses as a bonus.

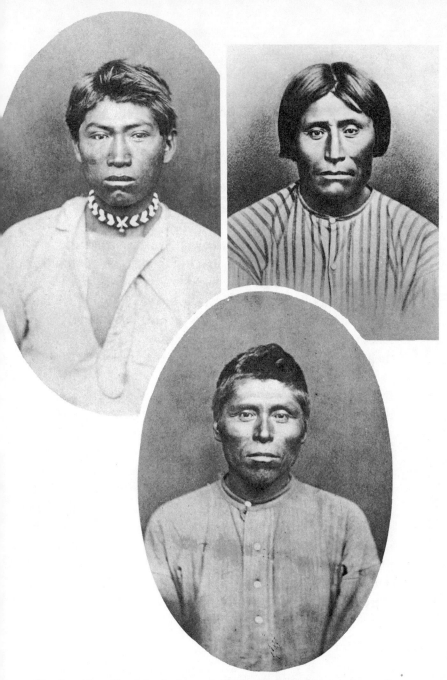

Hooker Jim, Captain Jack, and Curly Headed Doctor were the
leaders of the Modoc war in 1873. (*National Archives*)

The army had decided that it must warn other tribes from the path chosen by the Modoc. A well-publicized execution was thought to be a good policy. The newly elected President Grant decided to commute the sentence of two of the condemned to imprisonment because both the Indians and the military considered the youths to be below average intelligence and not fully responsible for their actions. But his mercy was kept secret until the very moment of execution on October 3, 1873, when Captain Jack and three others were hanged. The story of the Modoc resistance and the subsequent hangings swept the Indian nations. Rather than closing an era of conflict, the Modoc campaign was a prelude to a new series of wars. The policy of intimidation by execution proved to have the opposite effect. Chiefs who might have surrendered thought it best to continue fighting because they feared they would share the fate of Captain Jack.

The reservation the Modoc had desired consisted of two thousand acres and was valued at no more than twenty thousand dollars. The lava beds they would have taken as a substitute were worth considerably less. The American government had not been generous enough to grant the modest Modoc request. The final cost had been the death of a brigadier general, seven officers, thirty-nine privates, sixteen volunteers, two scouts, and eighteen civilians in a war costing more than half a million dollars. The humiliation was all the greater since the Modoc lost only five warriors, two of whom died examining an unexploded shell after a battle. The Modoc resistance was an affair the army wanted to forget as rapidly as possible. A magician more gifted than Curly Headed Doctor was needed to justify the bloody folly.

ISHI, LAST OF THE YAHI

One of the headlines of 1911 carried the astounding story of the discovery of a living "prehistoric" man in California. The individual was a starved Indian who had staggered into the corral of a slaughter house. His hair had been burned off close to his scalp and his only clothing was a ragged canvas cape. He would eat and drink nothing during his first days among the whites. Deer thongs hung from his ears and a wooden plug was in the septum of his nose. Somehow a man from the Neolithic Age seemed to have stumbled into the twentieth century.

Attempts to communicate with the wild man were useless. Indians tried various tribal dialects and Mexicans employed different Spanish idioms but there was no response. The strange man might have remained in his frenzied isolation until death had it not been for Albert Kroeber of the University of California. Kroeber was an expert on the California tribes and he knew of stories concerning a wild group of Yahi people belonging to the Yana nation. The professor visited the jail where the Indian was being held. He brought along a list of Yana words and then began to pronounce them one by one. The strange man listened intently but seemed to understand nothing until half way through the list Kroeber pronounced the word for wood correctly. The Indian's eyes glowed as if he had been recalled from the dead. He

pointed to the wood of his cot and repeated *siwini*. From
that first word a friendship developed that would endure
for the rest of the Indian's life and would reveal one of the
most pathetic stories concerning the white assault on
Native Americans.

The Yana people, made up of three to four thousand
people, lived in a mountainous region of California. The
Yahi subgroup to which the man of 1911 belonged had
about four hundred warriors. All the Indians of America
had watched the wagons moving westward, but the Yana
in California were among those who received the brunt
of land-hungry settlers who had crossed a continent of
miles to build new lives. Many of the Yana lived in back-
water regions, but their remoteness did not save them.
The best lands were soon taken and the whites sought
any fertile spot even if it were not of the first quality.
Adding to the difficulties of the Yana was the aggressive
spirit of the settlers. Land counted for everything and
Indian rights were nothing. Many of the men who arrived
during the period of the Gold Rush were frustrated by
the lack of women, by corruption, and by the failure to
make an instant fortune. Desperation of every variety
flourished and the Yana were perfect scapegoats. Between
1852–67 almost all the tribesmen became virtual slaves
of their white employers. Every Indian girl and woman
was subjected to being assaulted repeatedly or being forced
to become a prostitute. During the twenty years following
the Gold Rush venereal disease infected 40 to 80 per cent
of various tribes. Other diseases such as measles, chicken-
pox, smallpox, malaria, tuberculosis, typhoid, dysentery,
influenza, and pneumonia killed off most of the Indian
population.

The Yana were overwhelmed by the horrors that had

burst upon them so unexpectedly. They were a people who had no weapons as such beyond their hunting equipment. The first white man to live in their territory never saw one of them although he noticed logs they used to cross creeks and frequently spotted their footprints. The Yana did not bother the settlers but the new settlers thought any land they could hold on to with force was rightfully theirs. Desperados and toughs in saloons and bunkhouses smoldered with all the frustrations of frontier California. They found outlets for their disappointments in persecution of the Indians. Their cruelty is clearly recorded in many diaries kept by whites. The saloon gangs thought it was good sport to take Indian girls from their white employers, assault them and kill them by smashing their skulls. Yana who worked for whites were frequently stopped and robbed of their wages after being beaten unconscious. The men for whom the Indians worked were disturbed by what the hoodlums did but they would not risk their own security to save their Indian employees. The Yana began to fight back and the Yahi proved to be their most able warriors. The struggle reached its climax in the sixties when the Yahi were responsible for the death of fifty settlers.

The white response to the Indians' defense of their lives and honor was a series of massacres aimed at eventual extermination of every Yahi. The tribe retreated to living in caves and tried to avoid all contact with whites. Their birth rate fell far below the death rate as war reduced them to a fraction of their former numbers. By 1872 the tribe had decided the best way to resist was not to resist at all. They would simply vanish. The number of Yahi still alive at this time is unknown but it could not have been great or the tribe would not have been able to conceal itself so successfully. For twelve years the Yahi ceased to exist. Their warriors stole no horses and took no supplies. Everyone was careful to leave no footprints or damaged arrows. Ashes were scattered and campfires cunningly concealed. The men fished with the noiseless harpoon and net; they hunted with the silent bow and arrow; and they trapped with the voiceless snare. The Indians avoided known paths and scaled canyon walls using ropes made of milkweed fiber. Their memory was erased from the minds of whites.

The tribe had dwindled to a handful of individuals by 1884 and the last adult hunter had died. Hunger never left them. The band was forced to take greater risks as new roads and ranches penetrated into the most distant regions. The survivors slaughtered a few calves and stole some sheep to fight off starvation. They robbed cabins of flour and uncanned food. Most whites assumed the thieves to be outlaws or adolescents, but in 1885 four Yahi were seen by a settler as they attempted to steal from one of his cabins. The man described the Indians as a young woman, an old man, and two young boys, one crippled. The settler had a rifle and could have taken all four as prisoners but he was so moved by their pathetic condition that he waved them away with hopes for good fortune. The Indians were on the brink of starvation at this time yet they were so grateful for the unusual kindness that later in the year the man returned to the cabin to find two beautiful Indian baskets had been left for him upon the table.

In 1894 the raids ended once more as the remnant of no more than a dozen Indians retreated to an area near Deer Creek. The survivors soon dwindled to a family of five headed by the man who came to be known as Ishi. The family was always cautious that the whites should not see them or follow their trail. Ishi had been a fugitive all his life. He had never yet known a woman and never would. He never knew the routine of normal Indian life and never would. He never knew the happiness of tribal living and never would. He had been victimized as few American Indians had. Yet Ishi loved the things of nature and would have been content if the whites had allowed his small family to live in peace.

Legends about the wild Yahi persisted but they seemed to have no basis in fact until a settler's cabin was broken into in 1906. Definite proof that the Indians actually existed came two years later when the naked Ishi, now in his thirties, was seen by two men as he fished in a stream with his spear. A group of whites went looking for the hunter and came upon the cabins the five had lived in for so long. Ishi's wrinkled and white-haired mother was found under a pile of skins. Her semiparalyzed legs were swollen. Rather than moving the whites to compassion, the dying woman's condition disgusted them. They took all the food and other things of value in the cabin and left. One of them was so ashamed of his conduct that he returned the next day only to find the woman had disappeared.

Ishi had seen the party of whites and had hidden himself. His sister, carrying an old man on her back, had moved through the woods toward some hiding places near Deer Creek. After the whites had finished their ransacking Ishi carried his mother to another refuge where she died just a few days later. Ishi searched for his sister everywhere but he was never to see her or the old man again. He imagined they had drowned in the creek or been eaten by a bear or mountain lion. For the next three years, from November 1908 to August 1911, Ishi lived alone. His diet grew worse and worse. His spirit sank. He felt death calling so chose to burst dramatically upon the whites, half

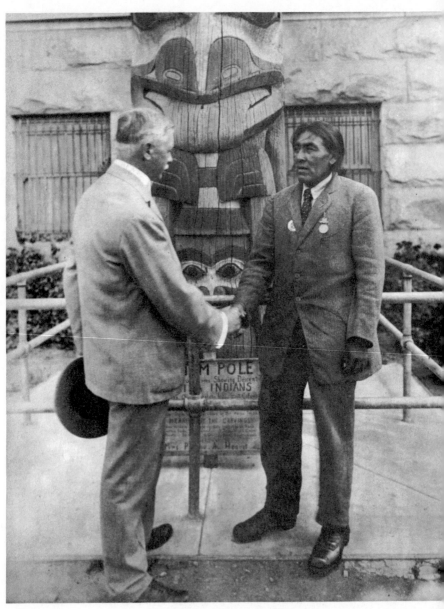

Ishi was teacher as well as student of the scholars who befriended him. (*Courtesy of Museum of the American Indian, Heye Foundation*)

wishing they would quickly put an end to the last of the Yahi.

The anthropologist who befriended Ishi at the jail took him to the Berkeley Museum in the "iron horse" Ishi's mother had said was a demon. At Berkeley, Ishi regained his health and came to know the men with whom he would share the remaining years of his life. The white professors were excited by the living history Ishi represented, but they also came to regard him as a personal friend. Ishi was given a room in the museum and he performed custodial tasks to earn money since no funds were given to him by the government or university in spite of the decades of brutalization the whites had subjected him to. Actually, Ishi was glad to work. He found everything in the white world new. The tools of the janitor were easier for him to cope with than the complex wonders of a twentieth-century city.

Men less idealistic than Kroeber and his colleague Thomas Waterman might have exploited Ishi as a cheap sideshow amusement, but the professors were of the best breed of whites. They developed their friend's self-esteem and confidence in whatever way they could. Ishi proved to have a generous soul and a quick mind. The learned anthropologists regarded him as a teacher as well as a student. Ishi understood the mutual nature of their relationship. He spent many of his days talking with them of Indian things or visiting with Dr. Pope, the university physician, who became one of his best friends. At specific hours, Ishi gave demonstrations of Indian lore to museum guests. Again, what might have become a sick spectacle was handled with such propriety that the children and adults who visited Ishi became appreciative learners rather than gawkers. Many of them returned frequently and some even corresponded with him from distant states.

Ishi enjoyed the enthusiasm of the whites, especially the children.

Ishi learned to use about six hundred English words and could carry on fairly complex conversations. He went about the city by himself and took trips with various friends. His reactions were often unpredictable. When taken to plays, he was more fascinated by the many whites sitting quietly row after row than by the entertainment on the stage. In 1914 a camping trip was made to the area around Deer Creek. At first, Ishi was filled with dread at the idea of returning to the place that had meant so much poverty and terror for him, but once back in the land he had grown to manhood in, his mood shifted. He felt happy to be close to nature once more and he demonstrated the ways his people had lived to the other men in the group. His confidence in his friends grew with each passing moon. He felt freer to tell more of his personal and tribal history. Many of his previous notions and taboos gave way before the common sense he found in what the whites taught. One thing he never revealed, however, was his true name. Ishi means man in Yana. Kroeber devised the name when pestered by newsmen about what to call him. The Indians of California were very reluctant to tell their names, for it conferred power over them to those who knew it. Ishi grew close to his white friends and probably would have told them his true name in time but as it was he died before such a confidence could be reached.

Ishi's grasp of the modern world progressed at a remarkable rate until his development was cut short by tuberculosis which struck him in late 1915 when he was approximately fifty-five years old. His illness was prolonged and the professors did all in their power to make him as comfortable as possible. Feeling he would be simply another patient in the hospital, his friends cleared out a wing of the museum and transformed it into a bedroom. Ishi was given constant attention and never lost his good cheer. Doctor Pope was at his side when Ishi finally died on March 25, 1916. The anthropologists were concerned that their friend's religious beliefs about the sanctity of the body after death be honored. Kroeber wrote to his colleagues, "If there is any talk about the interest of science, as for me, science can go to hell. We propose to

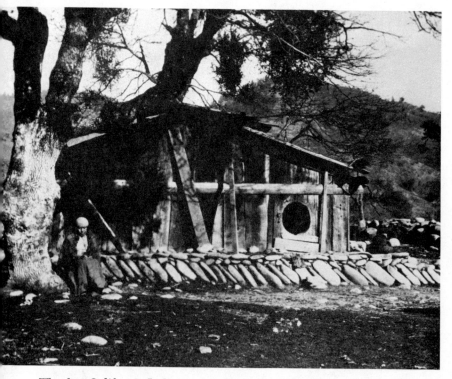

The few California Indians who survived mission life, disease, and war developed a life style very different from the simplicity of their traditional ways. (*Courtesy of Museum of the American Indian, Heye Foundation*)

stand by our friend." The state authorities thought otherwise and overruled such sentiments in order to have Ishi's brain preserved and an autopsy performed on his body. Ishi's death left Kroeber and Waterman deeply frustrated. They had only begun to explore with Ishi the traditions and skills of his nation. They had imagined they would have the leisure of a lifetime in which to learn from their unique and irreplaceable expert. A grief-stricken Waterman was despondent for years and called Ishi, "my best friend." Dr. Pope had had a more satisfying relationship with Ishi. Although they often discussed medical science with one another, their friendship flourished best when they fished and hunted together or when they compared the lore of the whites with that of the Indian. Pope saw deeply into the meaning of his friend's life and death when he wrote:

> And so, stoic and unafraid, departed the last wild Indian of America. He closed a chapter in history. He looked upon us as sophisticated children— smart, but not wise. We know many things, and much that is false. He knew nature, which is always true. His were the qualities of character that last forever. He was kind; he had courage and self-restraint and though all had been taken from him, there was no bitterness in his heart. His soul was that of a child, his mind that of a philosopher.

Part III

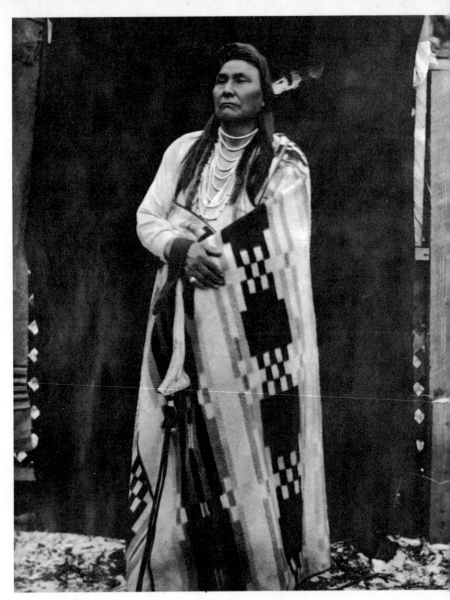

Chief Joseph of the Nez Percé helped lead a long unsuccessful fight for a reservation in Idaho, his homeland. He said, "I am tired of talk that comes to nothing. It makes my heart sick when I remember all the good words and all the broken promises." (*Courtesy of Museum of the American Indian, Heye Foundation*)

No More Forever:
THE NORTHWEST

I have only one heart. Although you say go to another country, my heart is not that way. I am here, and here is where I am going to be. I will not part with my lands. If you come again, I will say the same things. I will not part with my lands.

Unnamed Chief (Umatilla)

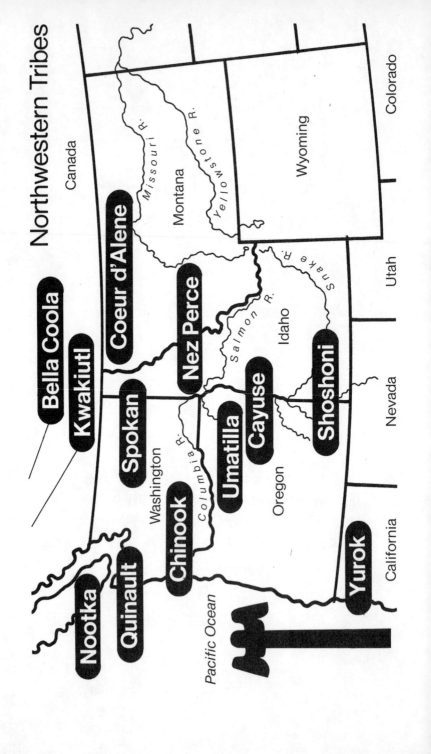

Northwestern Tribes

Canada

Bella Coola

Kwakiutl

Coeur d'Alene

Nez Perce

Spokan

Nootka

Quinault

Chinook

Washington

Columbia R.

Umatilla

Cayuse

Oregon

Shoshoni

Yurok

Pacific Ocean

Missouri R.

Montana

Yellowstone R.

Wyoming

Salmon R.

Snake R.

Idaho

Utah

Nevada

California

Colorado

POTLATCHERS AND TOTEM POLES

The salmon dominated the life of the Pacific Northwest as thoroughly as the buffalo dominated the life of the Great Plains. These fifteen-pound fish swimming up the rivers each summer and autumn were so numerous that early explorers bragged they could walk across the rivers on their backs. The oil-rich salmon meat was easily stored for use throughout the year and was the basic food of all tribes in the area. The ocean provided other food as well. Shellfish could be gathered on beaches, and each spring there were smelt thickly clustered on the surf. Spring also brought the oil-rich candlefish and herring which had the added advantage of leaving eggs that could be eaten at once. Farther out to sea were halibut, cod, sturgeon, sea otter, and sea lion. These fish could be taken by harpooning, spearing, dipnetting, and trapping. The Nootka of Vancouver Island even went out to the deepest waters to hunt the fifty-foot humpback whale from their rugged dugout canoes. Most important of all, however, were the salmon which sought to reproduce themselves in the quiet backwaters of the rivers emptying into the Pacific.

Like all the Indian nations, the tribes of the Pacific Northwest developed rituals to reconcile their belief in the sacredness of all life with their need to survive. They developed the idea that salmon were really spirits in special clothing. The first salmon of the year was taken by holy men and treated as a special visitor. The fish were thought to want to be caught and eaten, but their bones had to be returned to the water so that the salmon spirits could reclothe themselves for the following year. Exact rules were created for every act having to do with the salmon: catching, skinning, preparing, and eating.

The Northwest Indians were so prosperous that they developed a unique custom called the potlatch from the Nootka word *potshatl*, meaning *to give*. The potlatch was a feast in which an individual gained honor by giving away as many gifts as possible. Generosity, however, was not the motive of the gift giving, for each person who received a gift was under a strict obligation to make a return gift. Far from being a ceremony of sharing, the potlatch was an occasion for egotism and boasting which reinforced the prestige and power of the elite. The host worked hard to get acknowledgments of worth from his guests, and the guests worked hard to get gifts in keeping with what they felt they were owed. The potlatches were usually part of an important event such as marriage or the giving of a name. The gifts were a living symbol of the host's privileges and honors, and the giver let everyone know it:

> I am the only great tree, I the chief. I am the only great tree, I the chief. You here are right under me, tribes! You are my younger brothers under me, tribes! You surround me like a fence, tribes. I am your Eagle, the chief.

An important potlatch could take many years to arrange. First there was the process of accumulating the necessary items to be given away. This was followed by a diplomatic period during which representatives were sent to the various guests to work out the etiquette of the projected feast. The Quinault of Washington paid members of their own family to prepare the necessary food and paid other kinsmen to keep an account of what gifts the different guests should get and in what order they should be called on. The event itself had all the pageantry of a royal banquet. Guests were concerned about where they sat and in what order they were called to get their gifts, as well as in the quality and quantity of their gifts. *Everything* had to be eaten before the feast ended. When there was only one blanket left, the proud host placed it over his arm and asked, "Who will take it?" The guest who responded was taking responsibility for staging the next potlatch.

A rich man could rarely afford to give more than a few full-scale potlatches during his entire lifetime. The immediate effect of the event was to bankrupt him, although in time he would regain everything with interest at other potlatches where he was a guest. After the coming of the whites, the potlatches were increasingly influenced by their practices such as gifts having to be paid with interest. The decrease in Indian population because of disease also meant hereditary wealth accumulated on fewer individuals. The increasingly spectacular potlatches became wasteful exercises in ego with property and even human life destroyed to display wealth and power. These later potlatches with their accompanying abusive language have obscured the origins of the custom. The Kwakiutl of Vancouver Island speak of potlatches as wars of property rather than wars of blood. Fighting with goods and words seemed a vast improvement over spears and arrows. If two individuals were in competition for a bride or a title, they might stage rivalry potlatches rather than going to war. One Kwakiutl commented, "Now we fight with buttons, blankets, and other kinds of property. Oh, how good is the new time." The potlatchers also had play potlatches in which people laughed over the excessive language and imaginary gifts. Certainly the original potlatch custom had some of this feeling as well. The potlatches and gift giving also served to reward desired behavior patterns, especially among the young.

During the height of the potlatch fever, many minor gift-giving occasions were demanded of men of wealth. Again this is similar to the modern capitalist who must give generous tips to retain his popularity. A potlatcher had influence only so long as he had wealth he was willing to give away. His own artistic skills and knowledge were unimportant as long as he had the means to hire specialists. His gifts were a mixture of salaries, tips, loans, and bribes. An important man was also obliged to make up for social mishaps and disgraces with face-saving gifts or potlatches. So these fishing societies concentrated on the ability to gain riches. A successful person was thrifty and industrious. Marriages were planned as if they were business transactions. The man looked to increase his privileges and a woman sought a man who was as prestigious as possible as her worth was realized through his potlatches. Very much like the hardworking Puritans of New England, the potlatch people were taught to eat moderately and to work hard.

Wealth came in many forms. Dried fish, fine furs, and fish oil were basic, as were created objects such as canoes, blankets, baskets, and jewelry. The potlatchers had no money as such, but they used blankets, dentalia, and copper plaques as substitutes. Blankets were accumulated by the thousands and were handed out as small change. Dentalia were special conical sea shells fished up by the Nootka and placed on strings of special lengths. Whites who

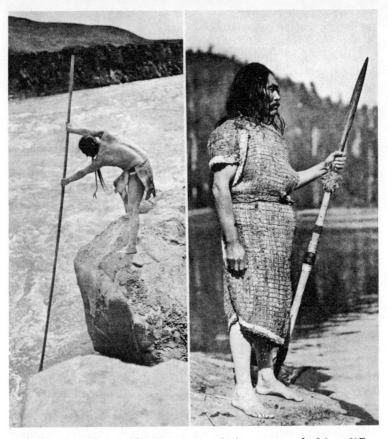

Fishermen of the northwest coast and rivers wore clothing different from most native North Americans and were among the minority of tribes to grow mustaches. (*Huntington Free Library, Heye Foundation*)

thought dentalia money found in the sea was silly were reminded by Indians that the yellow metal they prized could be found in the bottom of streams or in the earth. The Yurok of California decorated the dentalia with carvings and feathers and made it precise lengths. They were so possessed with the idea of accumulating it that their males were taught to have it constantly on their minds. Like some cartoon burlesque of a striver, they would awake at night shouting to the spirits that they wanted to be rich. They could be heard screaming aloud, "I want dentalia." The most prestigious signs of wealth, however, were copper plates of a foot to three feet in length. These were often decorated with designs, and their use meant the occasion was extremely serious. They became more and more valuable as they were traded. Originally, they had been associated with ancestor regard and were called "bones of the dead." Some coppers were given individual names and were protected from destruction as many coppers were broken in intense rivalry potlatches.

The lush forests provided yet another kind of wealth. Redwood and red cedar were easily carved. Northwest craftsmen made dugout canoes, houses, and utensils of all kinds. The canoes were carved directly from tree trunks and could be over thirty feet long. They were made without nails by simple animal tooth and stone tools, yet they could handle the roughest seas. The rectangular plank houses of the fishing societies were equally well built. They might extend for a hundred feet and often had slatted windows like modern Venetian blinds. Potlatchers also used wood to make everything from bowls to cradles and coffins.

Their most impressive artistic achievements were their totem poles and house façades. The first poles were seen by whites in 1794 and the art reached its peak in the hundred years which followed. The totem poles were not worshiped and they did not depict gods. Like most potlatcher customs, the totem building was a tribute to an owner's name. The poles told of a claim to being descended from the time of creation or to having a special relationship with the spiritual prototype of important animals. They symbolized the history of a family much as the heraldry, crests, and flags of the European medieval societies did. Fights over the merits and heights of poles became the cause of feuds. More than one killing stemmed from a villager raising a totem higher than that of his neighbor. Despite the nastiness sometimes surrounding them, the stunning totems and carved façades were sculpturing feats unrivaled in North America.

Economics tended to make the structure of potlatch societies rigid. The democracy and harmony that prevailed in most Indian societies were absent. There were nobles, commoners, and slaves. The nobles had special dances and privileges which they claimed went back "to the dawn of the world." But it was their wealth alone that gave them power. A chief's daughter would brag, "I am seated on coppers and have many names and privileges that will be given by my father to my future husband." Even cradle songs were tied to wealth. A boy child would be told, "Don't sleep, your paddle will fall into the water and your spear too. Don't sleep, for the ravens and cranes are flying away." A girl child would be told, "Don't sleep too much. Your digging stick will fall into the water and your basket. Wake up! It is nearly low water. You will be late going down to the beach."

Commoners might occasionally become rich if they were extremely industrious, talented, or lucky. Their best hope to advancement was to be in the service of a rich relative. An individual who had a striking vision or a skill in war or carving might attract the favor of a rich kinsman. Visions were critical, for without them a youth would not be taught a skill. Visionless young men often spent the night in terrifying places or scratched themselves bloody with thorns to bring on a dream. A rich youth usually dreamed of his favorite rich relative or the society he wanted to join. Commoners had ordinary visions and slaves rarely dreamed at all. A woman who

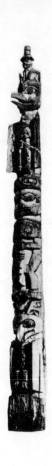

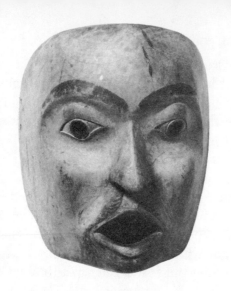

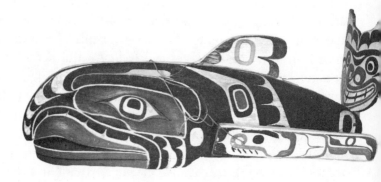

The people of the Northwest were among the world's greatest wood sculptors. The Bella Bella made the death mask, the Kwakiutl made the mechanical, potlatch mask, and the Tlingit made the totem pole. (*Courtesy of Museum of the American Indian, Heye Foundation*)

dreamed became a shaman.

Slaves had no chance to advance, for they were property and were treated as such, even being killed at some potlatches as an ultimate show of waste. Most slaves were women, and the Indian Puritans kept them healthy so that they could do all the routine and dull work. Although slaves could be bought, they were usually taken in raids. They might be stolen back or ransomed, but a face-saving potlatch was a must. Some nobles preferred to let their family members remain in captivity rather than go to the expense of a face-saving potlatch. Among the Yurok, a man could volunteer for slavery to pay off his debts, but men were usually not enslaved because they tried to escape and planned serious retaliations.

Even war was affected by the potlatch mentality. Some fights were agreed upon in advance, but most were in the form of surprise raids. The night before an attack, each warrior took omens to see how his luck was. A death warning or bad sign of any sort was sufficient grounds for a volunteer to dismiss himself with no loss of honor. The raids were often followed by peace negotiations where the potlatch rules came into their own. Neutral bargainers came from each side to go over the details of every killing, injury, and property damage with all the vigor of modern lawyers and insurance agents. Ceremonial and ritual damages were counted as equal to "real" damages. The Yurok fed their love of dentalia by making a payment necessary for every offense from trespassing to premeditated murder. Rather than an absolute value for injuries, there was a sliding scale with the penalty adjusted to the guilty one's ability to pay. This made for a lot of discussion and haggling, which the potlatchers liked. The rights of injured nobles were considered more important than those of commoners, which added yet another opportunity for establishing status.

Potlatch women were viewed as producers of wealth for their men. A noble might have many wives who worked hard themselves and who saw that their slaves were industrious in picking fruit, finding shellfish, weaving blankets, drying fish, and making baskets. Divorce was rare because of the required face-saving potlatch. During adolescence a girl must go into isolation for as long as a year in order to perform rituals and observe taboos. The rationale for this was that her suffering guaranteed future riches. Young women were constantly chaperoned and were expected to remain virgins. A lullaby from the northern tribes painted a rather glum picture for why women were born at all:

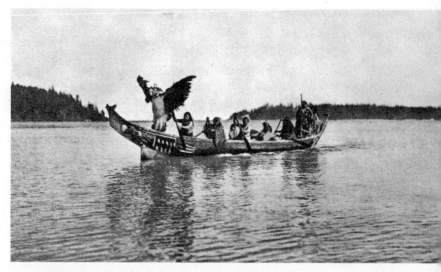

In order to insure a good salmon catch, ceremonies like this one were performed by the coastal people. (*Huntington Free Library, Heye Foundation*)

The little girl will pick wild roses.
That is why she was born.

The little girl will dig wild rice with her fingers.
That is why she was born.

She will gather sap of pitch pine trees in the spring.
She will pick strawberries and blueberries.
That is why she was born.

She will pick soapberries and elderberries.
She will pick wild roses.
That is why she was born.

When the Europeans began to sail into the area in the 1740s, the potlatchers entered a new era of wealth. Hundreds of ships called between 1774 and 1800. Their crews included many Chinese, Hawaiians, and Filipinos, who taught the Indians new carving skills. Many new products such as nails made life much easier. The whites took otter furs and other skins which they used to trade for the valuables of the Far East. The Indians called the beautiful Yankee clipper ships "Bostons" and their British counterparts were "King Georges." The greed of the potlatchers now fed on the goods the ships brought. Totem poles found new heights. Carvings were more skillful. Brass replaced stone. Guns and steel traps replaced harpoons, bows, and spears. The most profound change came with the establishment of the Hudson's Bay Company trading post in a place near present-day Seattle.

The gray blankets of the Hudson's Bay Company became so common they were a new currency. Few Indians bothered now with weaving blankets from animal skin or hair. Even fewer clung to the established patterns of animal conservation their fathers had taught them. The whites wanted furs and the whites were willing to pay well for them. The Indians felt released from traditional beliefs. Under the protection of the white man's magic, they hunted for hundreds of miles around the fort. They soon wiped out all the game just as the whites would one day wipe away almost all the salmon. They discarded the wisdom accumulated by their nations over the ages. In their frantic rush for wealth, they committed suicide.

Formal potlatches reached absurd proportions because there were far too many goods to be useful. Potlatches became more frequent and were grand displays of waste. Families were living extravagantly just to impress their neighbors. Populations dwindled as the white diseases struck. People like the Chinook disappeared entirely. Noble families died out. Commoners joined the crew of a ship and returned with more money than the most prosperous chiefs of old.

The system crashed into oblivion with the opening of the Oregon Trail in 1842. Within ten years, Oregon and Washington would be territories of the United States, California would have a Gold Rush, and the potlatchers would learn about reservations. Some tribes fought militarily but the groups were too small and scattered. Most of them found it easier to adapt to the new system and were more at ease within it than any previous Indian people had been. The transition was not without pain, however, and a Nootka song about the perpetual rain clouds could be given a new interpretation:

> Don't you ever,
> you up in the sky,
> don't you ever get tired
> of having clouds between you and us?

The potlatchers were a strange people with many disagreeable characteristics, but they were Indians and they placed importance on spiritual values. They had great respect for the dead and put much faith in shamans and the salmon spirits. Women were often shamans, and in some tribes only women could be shamans. The most impressive religious rituals took place in the forest. The Indians believed that in the beginning, creation had been put into order by a power related to one of the more clever creatures such as Raven or Mink. Dramatic dancing and feasting retold the creation myth as the Indians used grotesque masked figures to inspire and frighten one another. During these ceremonies, shamans might be possessed and be taken in a dream to Wolf or Salmon Village, where the spirits taught them arts to aid their people. The villagers danced to honor animal spirits, and the campfires often cast strange forest shadows as the skillful masked dancers acted out the exploits of Wolf or Cannibal Monster. Within their own value systems, the Northwesterners created a theater/religious event on the same artistic level as the more widely known efforts of the Pueblo.

Much has been written about the unpleasant, vain, and materialistic nature of the fishing people, especially in comparison to the gentle Pueblo. It is almost as if the whites were shocked to see their own values apparently mocked in such a stark fashion. But the potlatchers were very much concerned with traditional Indian spiritual values. Chief Seattle of the Suquamish and Duwamish addressed a warning to the whites of the state of Washington in 1855 which is one of the most eloquent of all Indian speeches:

> Your religion was written upon tables of stone by the iron finger of your God so that you could not forget. The Red Man could never comprehend nor

remember it. Our religion is the traditions of our ancestors—the dreams of our old men, given to them in the solemn hours of night by the Great Spirit; and the visions of our sachems and is written in the hearts of our people.

Your dead cease to love you and the land of their nativity as soon as they pass the portals of the tomb and wander way beyond the stars. Our dead never forget the beautiful world that gave them being . . .

A few more moons. A few more winters—and not one of the descendants of the mighty hosts that once moved over this broad land or lived in happy homes, protected by the Great Spirit, will remain to mourn over the graves of a people—once more powerful and hopeful than yours. But why should I mourn at the untimely fate of my people? Tribe follows tribe, and nation follows nation, like the waves of the sea. It is the order of nature, and to regret it is useless. Your time of decay may be distant, but it will surely come, for even the White Man whose God walked and talked with him as friend with friend cannot be exempt from the common destiny. We may be brothers after all. We will see.

. . . Every part of this soil is sacred in the estimation of my people. Every hillside, every valley, every plain and grove has been hallowed by some sad or happy event in days long vanished. Even the rocks, which seem to be dumb and dead as they swelter in the sun along the silent shore, thrill with memories of stirring events connected with the lives of my people, and the very dust upon which you now stand responds more lovingly to their footsteps than to yours, because it is rich with the blood of our ancestors and our bare feet are conscious of the sympathetic touch . . . And when the last Red Man shall have perished, and the memory of my tribe shall have become a myth among the White

Men, these shores will swarm with the invisible dead of my tribe, and when your children's children think themselves alone in the field, the store, the shop, upon the highway, or in the silence of the pathless woods, they will not be alone. In all the earth there is no place dedicated to solitude. At night when the streets of your cities and villages are silent and you think them deserted, they will throng with the returning hosts that once filled and still love this beautiful land. The White Man will never be alone.

Let him be just and deal kindly with my people, for the dead are not powerless. Dead, did I say? There is no death, only a change of worlds.

THE LONGEST MARCH

All the people of the plateau made the journey from good will to hatred for the whites, but the Nez Percé rode the saddest trail of all. They lived east of the potlatchers in the valleys of the Clearwater, the Salmon, and the Snake rivers. In this region where Washington, Oregon, and Idaho meet there were deep canyons, ridges, and evergreen forests. The valleys ranged in width from virtually nothing as in the case of famous Hell's Canyon to narrow bottomlands from one half to three fourths of a mile wide. Beyond the canyons were hills and occasional flat or rolling prairies. The seasons were clearly defined. Summer meant grasses and flowering prairies, while winter brought biting frost and deep snows. The Nez Percé land was not well suited to the interests of the whites but the tall regal people prized their valleys above all things known beneath the sky.

Salmon was the main food of the Nez Percé and permanent settlements existed near the best streams which were recognized as the territory of specific bands, but deer, bear, and mountain sheep provided variety in Nez Percé diets. The American horse had become extinct in prehistoric times, but the Europeans had brought horses with them, and the Nez Percé loved the new animal very much. They became among the most skillful tribes not only in handling horses but in breeding and trading them. Horses allowed the Nez Percé to travel and hunt much easier than before. They began to use the western edge of the plains for buffalo hunting and adopted many of the habits of the people of the plains. The other salmon-eating Indians called the Nez Percé "horse Indians" to mark them off from the salmon eaters on the coast who traveled mainly on foot or by canoe.

Lewis and Clark entered the Nez Percé and Shoshone country in 1806 as part of their exploration of the Louisana Purchase. The explorers had a young Shoshone woman with them whose reunion with her tribe created immense good will for the Americans, but such good will was only an extension of the usual hospitality for strangers. The Nez Percé were always noted for treating traders and visitors with kindness. The white men who came up the great rivers wanted to trade their products for the things of the forest, an arrangement which left Indian life pretty much as the whites had found it. A new prosperity swept the region but the awful price was the killing diseases of the whites that came up the same rivers as the trading canoes. Along the main routes of trade, people such as the Chinook, who had always been among the most eager to barter, became extinct. The scourge of 1831 was smallpox, but each year a new disease came to take heavy tolls, with cholera which killed thousands in 1849 being among the worst. The Nez

Percé were alarmed by this march of death and when they heard of a Holy Book whose magic was mightier than anything else the whites possessed they were anxious to have its protection. In 1831 they sent a delegation one thousand miles to speak with their friend Clark who was living in St. Louis. The explorer was sympathetic toward their desire for the new religion, but he said he could not agree to sending missionaries when the new trail was still so dangerous. Only one of the Nez Percé travelers survived the return trip. He told his people that Rabbitskin Leggings, the leader of the delegation, had told Clark: "I came with one eye partly opened. I sought light. I return with both eyes shut and my arms broken."

In less than ten years the formidable thousand miles of dangerous trail became a crowded roadway bringing not one set of reluctant missionaries but many competing groups. Marcus Whitman was the first to establish a permanent white settlement. He opened the Oregon Trail in 1841–42 and welcomed a thousand travelers the next year. The new whites were not loners who came by mule or canoe but entire families loaded with housewares, tools, children, and livestock. Their heavy prairie schooners cut deep ruts into the soil as they took weeks to cross the rivers of the West before resting in safety at Fort Hill. Eventually they pushed on to Fort Boise and from there to the Columbia River, which took them to the fertile territories of Washington and Oregon. By 1852, the settlers were passing through at the rate of ten thousand a year.

These first waves of immigration did not disturb the Nez Percé. The travelers were too anxious to reach the valleys beyond the mountains to consider stopping in the difficult country with the harsh winters. Many tribes were so unconcerned about the whites that they actually helped them cross dangerous rivers and collected stray cattle for them. Some joked about the pale faces of the strangers, but many of them never saw a white at all. Yellow Wolf of the Nez Percé would remember these days with fondness. He spoke of the mountains, springs and running waters "of my own country when only Indians were there. Of tepees along the bending river. Of the blue clear lake, wide meadows with horse and cattle herds. From the mountain forests, voices seemed to be calling. I felt as dreaming."

The tribes of Washington and Oregon had different attitudes. The valleys the whites desired were their homelands. Wars broke out with increasing fury and frequency. The Indians fought so well that most of the settlements were closed down, but the victory was only momentary. Soon, fresh waves of immigrants with new types of rifles came down the Columbia. Tribes such as the Spokane and Coeur d'Alene which had never fought before took up arms. The Nez Percé were urged to join the struggle, but they refused. They even protected whites when the Marcus Whitman Mission fell to the Cayuse, who had always been friends and neighbors. The Nez Percé thought of themselves as peaceful and reasonable folk. They could not imagine why there should ever be war between them and the United States.

Some of the Nez Percé adopted the Christian religion or wove parts of it into their traditional faiths, but a large number remained loyal to the Dreamer Cult, which stressed the sacred nature of the earth. Chief Joseph the Younger explained some of the cult's basic beliefs to a white commission:

> [The Creative Power] was made of the earth and grew up on her bosom. The earth was his mother and nurse and was sacred to his affection . . . More-over the earth carried chieftainship . . . and there-

fore to part with the earth would be to part with himself or his self-control.

Toohulhulsote, one of the chief advocates of the Dreamer Cult, said, "The earth is part of my body." Such attachment to the land led the Nez Percé to be careful about making any treaties, but the Dreamer faith went beyond generalized nature worship to instill moral virtues. Chief Joseph the Younger explained that the Nez Percé were taught that they should never be the first to break a bargain, that it was a disgrace to tell a lie, and that a great spirit saw and heard everything on earth. Early settlers remarked that when Nez Percé were witnesses at trials they refused to hold up their hand and take an oath because they spoke the truth all the time.

These truthtellers so attached to the earth called themselves Nimpau—the real people. The name Nez Percé most likely stemmed from a time in their past when they had worn ornaments in their noses, a practice they had given up by the time of Lewis and Clark. The tribe was always noted for its passive nature but as the 1850s wore on, the whites demanded treaties. In 1855 the head men reluctantly agreed to give up some land with the guarantee that all the remaining valleys would remain Indian for "as long as the grass shall grow and the water flow." The matter seemed settled until 1861 when gold was discovered on Nez Percé land. A new agreement was negotiated, temporarily opening additional lands for mining. Two years later the whites demanded more land and the chiefs, who had been hesitant before, refused to sign away any more territory. The councils of the Nez Percé met and the tribe divided into three equal factions.

The group that would come to be called the Treaty Nez Percé agreed to sign the new treaty because the land to be given up was not part of their territory even though they would share in the gifts which came with the agreement. A second group absolutely refused to consider giving up any more land. The third block regretted having signed any treaties and demanded that the lands already given up be returned. Among the nonsigners were Looking Glass the Elder and Joseph the Elder. These head men had been wary about signing in the first place for they understood that he who has the right to give also has the right to take away. The whites had no valid claim to their land. Joseph believed that no man owned any part of the earth and thus no man could sell any part of it. The signatures of the Treaty Nez Percé could no more bind the entire nation than one third of the Senate could bind the United States. But the Indian Bureau had long made it official policy to accept such convenient absurdities as justice. Those who would not go on reservations they had never agreed to go on and would not give up land they had never agreed to give up were termed "hostiles." Only the shock of the Civil War and the remoteness of the Nez Percé region allowed the dispute to remain unsettled. Old Joseph was so disgusted with the whites he tore up a Bible he had possessed for thirty years and vowed he would no longer have anything to do with the whites.

Not a summer passed from that time on when an army agent or a spokesman for the Indian Bureau did not attempt to persuade the Non-Treaties to accept reservations. At the close of the Civil War more whites moved west and they began to settle in the plateau region in greater numbers than before. The Nez Percé prepared summaries of their positions and sent them to Washington, D.C. President Grant was so impressed by the merits of their arguments that in 1873 he signed an executive order returning half the land the Non-Treaties had never signed away. Idaho whites became so enraged over the President's decision that their political representatives were able to get it reversed in less than two years. The chiefs who had refused to sign died but in their places were Looking Glass the Younger and Joseph the Younger, two shrewd and able leaders whose abilities matched their patriotism.

The fatal hour for the Non-Treaties struck in 1877. The Modoc to the south had fought their incredible war only a few years before and the Sioux to the east had annihilated Custer the previous summer but the United States still thought it could handle the Nez Percé roughly. The tribe had never fought whites. They were famous for their good sense and co-operation. The orders went out that they must go to a reservation immediately or the army would arrest them. General Howard made the ultimatum unnecessarily cruel by posting a thirty-day limit for the surrender. The herds and villages of the Non-Treaties were widely scattered. If they were to reach the designated spot on a nearby prairie by the deadline of June 15, they had to cross the formidable Snake and Grand Ronde rivers. Howard would find crossing the rough waters a terrible ordeal for his own tough soldiers just a few weeks later but at this point he expected families to transport all their possessions and numerous animals over the rivers in a relatively short space of time.

Both Joseph and Looking Glass had chosen to comply. The Nez Percé head men were not foolish. They realized they could not win an armed struggle with the United States. General Howard's ultimatum might well have succeeded except for some of the younger warriors. The Nez Percé had been peaceful Indians but as always in relations between Indians and whites there were a number of unpunished murders on both sides which made violence possible at any time. Earlier, Howard had imprisoned Too-

hulhulsote for insolence and for insisting on the traditional
Nez Percé customs. Now the army wanted to take all the
Non-Treaty land. The white chief was making the tribes
lose valuable livestock by forcing them to cross treacherous
rivers at a difficult time of the year. If the Nez Percé head
men were old women who feared death, there were at least
three young braves who would defend the honor of the
nation, avenge the dead, and protect the beliefs of the
Dreamers. The self-styled heroes put on their war paint
and began a series of raids which resulted in a dozen
dead whites.

The news of the killings came to Joseph's band while it
was still trying to comply with Howard's demands. The
chief understood at once that the army might not be overly
careful about locating exactly which braves in which
band had committed the murders. Joseph decided to move
his people to White Bird Canyon to await developments.
Within a short time, other groups of Non-Treaties began
to join him. The chiefs did not approve of what their
young warriors had done but they would not give them up
to the inconsistencies of white justice. Many killers of their
own people had gone unpunished.

Looking Glass had not joined the outbreak. He sent
word to his neighbors not to go near his lodges and involve
his group in their "useless and foolish struggle." Joseph
and the other men debated on the possibility of making
some sort of bargain with the angry whites, but a force
of one hundred army volunteers cut short their council.
The whites imagined they could score an easy victory as
the Nez Percé had no reputation as fighting men. These
volunteers became the first to discover that the Nez Percé
were the finest marksmen of all the Indians with an un-
usually good sense of tactics. A handful of Nez Percé approached the whites under a truce flag but they were im-

mediately fired upon and forced to take cover to save their lives. The whites charged valiantly but within a short time a third of them were dead and the seventy warriors who had dropped them were chasing the survivors across the canyon floor.

The Nez Percé were elated with their easy triumph, but they were divided over future tactics. The various points of view discussed at the White Bird councils would be repeated throughout the course of the war which followed. Joseph wanted to stay in the valley and fight. Either the whites would be persuaded to let them have a reservation in their old territories or the Nez Percé would perish defending their one true homeland. Others argued that they should move to the land of the Crow which was out of General Howard's department. The whites in other regions would have no reason to persecute them. Still others thought it best to unite with the Sioux in an intertribal confederation for survival. The Nez Percé had never fought against whites before but they had already won the first battle of a running war that would carry them through more than one thousand miles of enemy soldiers, cultivated valleys, and wildernesses. They would win any number of skirmishes with the military yet retain enough discipline to spare civilian populations. The talking wires would carry news of their heroic struggle to the entire United States and perhaps for the first time in North American history there would be many whites who wished Indians some sort of victory.

Upon hearing of the White Bird Canyon debacle General Howard ordered his troops to march against the Nez Percé. He foolishly complicated his task by sending a detachment to round up the band of Looking Glass. Making no effort to determine the mood of the band, the troops attacked the unguarded camp as if it were the center of Nez

Percé resistance. The toll in families and warriors was high but the majority of the band fled to safety. When the angered tribesmen regathered they decided to join the hostiles rather than submit to such brutal intimidation. Looking Glass became one of the major war leaders of the united hostiles, and his braves would seek revenge for their slain relatives in many future battles. While Howard's detachment was busy creating such substantial new enemies, his main body of three hundred men accomplished nothing. The hostiles had left White Bird Canyon and thrown Howard off their trail by crossing and recrossing the Salmon River. On July 3 an army scouting party of ten was wiped out by Nez Percé ambushers. The army began its painful re-evaluation of Nez Percé bravery and military ability.

The Non-Treaties made their new camp on the Clearwater River and thereby committed their first and only major error of the campaign. If they were to achieve success against the army they needed to remain mobile but at Clearwater the bands set up a semipermanent camp. They had the foresight to build defensive rifle pits, a device which characterized all future camps, but other than that the Indians made no preparations to defend themselves. Their strength had grown to two hundred warriors and four hundred women, children, and aged.

The Nez Percé scouts had spotted every previous army move but on July 11, Howard surprised the camp. His force was made up of four hundred regulars, two hundred volunteers, and assorted units of artillery. Even with surprise added to his overwhelming numerical advantage, he was not able to overrun the Nez Percé positions. The rifle pits with their rock protection were well placed and precise marksmanship drove the attackers back. The following day a fresh assault found the camp deserted. The casualties in the battle were few. Howard lost thirteen killed and twenty-seven wounded. He estimated that the Nez Percé lost twice as many although the Indians would only admit four killed and six wounded when questioned after the war. The significance of the battle was not in the loss of life but in the destruction or capture of almost all of the considerable possessions of the Nez Percé. Joseph would write that Howard broke him upon the Clearwater, and white historians refer to the battle as the Gettysburg of the Nez Percé. The nation had been wealthy and it was a hard blow to lose everything in a single battle, but the Nez Percé still retained their fighting ability and determination to resist. Joseph was willing to fight a battle to the death in the valleys but the council decided it was best that the tribe move to buffalo country.

Howard pursued the fleeing Nez Percé to the banks of the Klamath River where his force was held off by a rear guard of Nez Percé fighting men. The Indians now struck out across the treacherous Lolo Trail that led over the Bitterroot Mountains. Howard found it impossible to move with any speed along the route and telegraphed ahead for others to delay the Indians while he tried to catch up. At a gap in the mountains a barricade was hastily constructed by thirty soldiers and three hundred civilians. When the Nez Percé arrived at the barrier they told the civilians that their fight was not with them but with General Howard. They did not want to kill any whites and they certainly had no quarrel with the people of the Bitterroot Valley. If they were allowed free passage through the area they promised they would neither loot nor kill. The settlers knew the reputation of the Nez Percé and the Indian diplomats were so eloquent that the tribe was allowed to pass by the barricade that came to be remembered as Fort Fizzle. At towns in the valley the Indians made purchases of sugar, coffee, tobacco, and other goods with their remaining gold dust and greenbacks. Not all the young men could be restrained but the chiefs kept their word as much as possible. Their train sometimes stretched for as long as three miles and contained two to three thousand horses. The slight damage suffered by the people of Bitterroot was nothing compared to the deaths a battle at the gap would have entailed.

The Indians did not camp again until they reached a valley beyond the Continental Divide. They thought they would have time to rest and enjoy themselves, but they were mistaken. Colonel Gibbon had left Fort Shaw with orders to find them. He pushed his men day and night, and when scouts brought word of the Nez Percé camp, he rushed to attack. During the first moments of the charge, it seemed the Indians were about to suffer a defeat surpassing the one upon the Clearwater. White Bird and Looking Glass happened to be isolated at opposite ends of the camp by the attack. Soon their strong voices rallied the stunned Nez Percé warriors. The Indian rout suddenly turned into its opposite. Gibbon's men fell back in panic shouting that they had been trapped in the same manner Custer had been trapped. The Indian counterattack was so sweeping that the warriors even captured Gibbon's cannon. If the Nez Percé had known how to use artillery, Gibbon's men would have been pounded to death by their own guns. Joseph's role in the actual fighting was slight as he had the responsibility of gathering up the supplies and leading the nonfighters to safety.

Gibbon gathered his men on high ground where Nez Percé rifle fire immobilized them. The main body of Indians returned to their camp to find that of the eighty-seven dead, seventy were women, children, and the old. Gibbon would write:

Few of us will soon forget the wail of mingled rage and horror which came from the camp four or five hundred yards from us when the Indians returned to it and recognized their slaughtered warriors, women, and children. Above this wail of horror we could hear the passionate appeal of the leaders urging their followers to fight and the war hoops in answer which boded us no good.

The warriors buried their dead and gradually filtered back to the rifle pits and again their deadly accuracy terrified the whites. The sharpshooters would undoubtedly have shot and starved Gibbon's men to death but word reached them that the plodding General Howard was approaching. The Nez Percé retreated, leaving the army with thirty-three dead and thirty-eight wounded. Howard was shocked when he came upon the destroyed Gibbon, as he had thought the Clearwater battle had meant the war was finished. His Bannock scouts had been promised horses. Their anger drove them to dig up the corpses of the dead Nez Percé to mutilate and scalp them. When the Nez Percé heard of this outrage they were horrified and their estimation of Howard's character diminished.

The new trails of the Nez Percé led them through Yellowstone National Park, which was just five years old. The Indians moved efficiently and quickly but many individuals took the opportunity to gaze at the spurting geysers of steam and the bubbling mudpits. The head men strove to control their young warriors, but several touring parties were harassed and two whites lost their lives. By a quirk of fate General Sherman, the chief of all the armies of the white nation, was visiting in the park. Sherman no more suspected the presence of the Nez Percé than they suspected his. The tribesmen would have been able to capture him easily had they been aware he was so near.

The tribe maneuvered cleverly. Their false trails and decoy herds were so effective that several sizable groups sent against them were thrown off the trail completely or hopelessly delayed. Looking Glass, White Bird, Toohulhulsote, Lean Elk, and Poker Joe were among the influential Nez Percé leaders. The success of the tribe was a group effort but the white newspapers spoke only of Joseph who was given sole credit for outwitting so many white adversaries.

The Indians came out of the park at Clark's Fork on the Yellowstone River. They met some Crow who were willing to give them supplies but could not harbor Non-Treaties because they were army scouts and had good relations with the whites. At this point the only alternative left to the Nez Percé was to cross to Canada and join Sitting Bull. Even though the Crow refused to scout against the Nez Percé, Major General Sturgis, commander of the reorganized 7th Regiment, learned about their location. Vigorous marches enabled the regiment to catch the Indians at their camp at Canyon Creek in Montana. The white pony soldiers were fatigued from their march, yet the Indians who had been on the march so much longer threw back their initial attacks easily. Not even a spirited charge by Custer's old regiment seeking desperately to restore its lost prestige could shake the Nez Percé defense. The Indians began to withdraw under the cover of darkness, and the weary cavalrymen had neither the will nor the resources to give pursuit.

What proved to be the last Nez Percé camp was pitched forty miles south of the Canadian border in the Bear Paw Mountains. The tribe had never fought whites until their homeland was demanded. Even in war they had shown an extraordinary discipline and honor that the various civilian and military units sent against them rarely equaled. They had maneuvered and fought as well as any tribe and they had overcome artillery, the talking wire, and continual fresh troops. They were willing to leave the United States forever, but the army would not allow them even that last comfort. Colonel Miles with Cheyenne scouts and six hundred fresh men steamed and marched 150 miles to attack them during the last days of September. He brought machine guns and cannon. Much of the camp was already packed for the final dash into exile when he struck.

Miles ordered a full mounted charge on the camp, thinking to smash resistance with one decisive blow. The Nez Percé had marched so far and suffered so many wounds, Miles assumed the warriors would snap. Such was not the case. The accurate Nez Percé rifle fire brought down 20 per cent of the advancing soldiers. Even if the charge had managed to capture the rifle pits, the casualty rate would have been considered high. As it was, the charge was a failure. Miles had to call retreat. A little over one hundred weary warriors had turned back one of the best trained cavalry units. Miles consoled himself with the thought that at least he had the Nez Percé trapped, but he soon wondered about that, too, as Nez Percé sharpshooters selected his officers as special targets. Snow began to fall. Miles was no longer certain whether he was besieger or the besieged.

The men under Miles fought back with courage equal to that of the Indians. The Nez Percé lost seventeen dead and more than forty wounded. Toohulhulsote, Poker Joe, Looking Glass, and other leaders were killed. The deaths of so many important men were disheartening, but the only two chiefs of major status left alive, Joseph and White Bird, would not surrender. They sent runners to Sitting Bull to ask his assistance.

The Nez Percé messengers never reached the Sioux medicine man. The Indians assumed that some Assiniboin killed them out of fear of being drawn into a new war with the whites. Other sources brought the news of the battle, and the Sioux wanted to ride to the rescue at once. The Canadian Northwest Mounted Police rode into camp to warn the Sioux that if they should recross the border to fight they would lose all rights of political asylum and sanctuary. While Sitting Bull's council meditated, Miles was suffering badly. In one group of 115 men, he had lost 53 killed or wounded. In other companies he had lost one third of his men with 40 more wounded. There were almost no facilities for tending the injured and the weather grew progressively worse. It was with relief that Miles discovered Joseph wanted to discuss possible peace terms. The chief came under a flag of truce and a reporter assigned to the army got his first glimpse of the Indian whose exploits had thrilled the whites of the United States:

> Physically Joseph is a splendid-looking man. He is fully six feet high; in the prime of life—about 35, has a splendid face and well-formed head. His forehead is high, his eyes bright yet kind, his nose finely cut, and his mouth though determined, rather too sad-looking for actual beauty.

Joseph was inclined to surrender but even with most of the other leaders dead he was still not in complete control of the Indian camp. Unable to reach a satisfactory agreement the chief was about to return to his own people when Miles had him seized. The colonel was frustrated by the faltering siege and the prospect that the thousand-mile campaign might yet end in failure. His treachery was not premeditated like the treachery of General Jesup with the Seminole chief Osceola but, though many thousands of miles and many thousands of days separated the cold of Montana from the sunshine of Florida, a white general again forsook his honor to arrest an Indian carrying a white truce flag. Joseph escaped the fate of his Seminole counterpart only because his own men happened to capture a white officer. An ashamed Miles was forced to trade his valuable "prisoner" for one of his subordinates.

On October 4 General Howard arrived to reinforce Miles. He had patiently stayed on the trail of the Nez Percé the entire distance from Idaho. The military situation was now hopeless for the Non-Treaties. Joseph was disturbed about the welfare of his people. Many of them were wandering helplessly in the mountains with little food and scant protection from the cold. His men were weak. There had been no word from Sitting Bull. The decision to go to Canada had been forced on them. The Nez Percé did not object to reservation life so much if they could have land in one of their old valleys. He had counseled peace at many meetings and now he offered to surrender if the whites would respect certain terms: his people must be cared for in Montana until spring when they could be returned to a reservation in the valleys of Idaho. After a brief consideration of Joseph's proposal, Miles and Howard agreed. Joseph responded with a surrender message that brought tears to the eyes of the Nez Percé interpreters and moved even the hardened military men by its stoic eloquence:

> Tell General Howard I know his heart. What he told me before I have in my heart. I am tired of fighting. Looking Glass is dead. Toohulhulsote is dead. The old men are all dead. It is the young who say yes or no. He who led on the young is dead. It is cold and we have no blankets. The little children are freezing to death. My people, some of them, have run away to the hills, and have no blankets, no food. No one knows where they

are, perhaps freezing to death. I want to have time to look for my children and see how many of them I can find. Maybe I shall find them among the dead. Hear me my chiefs, I am tired; my heart is sick and sad. From where the sun now stands I will fight no more forever.

The army men were astounded by the weak condition of the surrendering warriors. The formidable enemy who had eluded them over so many miles consisted mainly of hardy women and children protected by a few incredibly brave men. Howard had understood from the start that he was pursuing a band of families and not a war party but only in the moments of final surrender did he realize the problems the Indian chiefs had faced.

White Bird was so skeptical of white honor that he slipped away with his followers to the camp of Sitting Bull. The old chief spoke often of Captain Jack and thought that since the killers who started the outbreak were from his group he might be held responsible for their actions. He also doubted the whites would keep their pledge regarding a reservation in Idaho. Events proved White Bird correct.

The Nez Percé who surrendered were first taken to Bismarck, North Dakota, where the townspeople behaved as no white people had ever before behaved toward captured Indians. They presented the tribe with food and much needed clothing. They made no secret of their best wishes for the defeated Nez Percé. Such behavior proved to be the last translation of favorable public opinion into positive acts that the Nez Percé would experience. Miles wanted to keep his pledge but his superiors asserted that the peace terms were improper. The tribe was not taken to Montana but south to a military reservation at Fort Leavenworth, Kansas. Some time later the group was taken to a reservation in Oklahoma. In three agonizing years almost two hundred Nez Percé died and the rest were broken in health and spirit.

General Miles was appointed commander of the region containing Idaho in 1881. He wanted to honor his pledge to Joseph and wrote a letter to the President of the United States personally vouching for the Nez Percé character and documenting the cruelty of the Oklahoma confinement. Miles had married the daughter of a prominent senator and he was the in-law of General Sherman as well as being a famous Indian fighter in his own right. The President listened respectfully, but the residents of Idaho argued vigorously against the return of the "wild" Nez Percé. The Great White Father could not find the courage to risk political disfavor for the mere sake of justice or honoring a field agreement made by one of his most respected chiefs. He soothed his conscience by allowing the Nez Percé to be moved to Lapwai, a northern reservation. Almost at once the Presbyterian Mission there objected to having any Dreamers come to them. The Indian interpreters sent to speak with the Nez Percé asked, "Where do you want to go? Lapwai and be a Christian or Colville and just be yourself?" Joseph and most of his followers chose the Colville Reservation of the Spokane.

In the discussion which continued about the surrender, Joseph insisted he would have chosen death before giving up if Miles and Howard had not promised to return them to their homeland. The newspapers had depicted him as a red Napoleon, but he was simply a powerful voice in the councils of a people who tolerated no emperors. Even his personal fame and prestige were of no use in securing a reservation in the Wallowa Valley. People were impressed by his writings and speeches. They felt the emotion behind his simple statement, "I love that land more than all the rest of the world." But the government would not grant his one wish. It was not until 1900 that he was even allowed to visit his former home. The inspector who was required to go with him reported that the old warrior wept when he saw that a settler had taken care of his father's grave.

His own death came four summers later while he was sitting in contemplation before a fire. The agents at Colville listed "a broken heart" as the official cause of death. A former aide of General Howard would write, "I think in

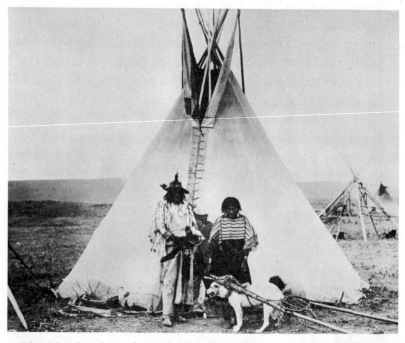

This Nez Percé couple, with their dog pulling a travois, might have been one of the families that followed Joseph on the long march from Idaho to North Dakota, only to end eventually on an Oklahoma reservation. (*Courtesy of Museum of the American Indian, Heye Foundation*)

all his long career, Joseph cannot accuse the government of the United States of a single act of justice." Certainly the fate of the Native Americans was clear to Joseph as he sat before the dying flame those last years. Soon Indians would be curiosities and amusements for the whites. They would be servants or beggars or worst of all, as Black Hawk of the Wisconsin Sauk had predicted, they would be just like the whites. The Nez Percé nation was dead even though Nez Percé bodies lingered. Perhaps one day the flesh of the Indian would perish altogether leaving only his soul to cast a red shadow in the dusk. Yet when his fire snapped loudly or unexpectedly flared brightly, Joseph would remember the teachings of his people. For a short time the man the Nez Percé knew as Hein-mot Too-ya-La-kekt could dream again:

> *You ask me to plow the ground.*
> *Shall I take a knife and tear my mother's breast?*
> *Then when I die*
> *She will not take me to her bosom to sleep.*
>
> *You ask me to dig for stone.*
> *Shall I dig under her skin for bones?*
> *Then when I die*
> *I cannot enter her body to be born again.*
>
> *You ask me to cut grass and make hay,*
> *And sell it and be rich like the white man.*
> *But how dare I cut off my mother's hair?*
>
> *It is a bad law and my people cannot obey it!*

INDEX

NOTE: *Page numbers in boldface refer to illustrations.*